Renate Klein is Lecturer in Women's Studies at Deakin University. She is a biologist, member of FINRRAGE and author/editor of numerous books on reproductive technologies, Women's Studies and feminist theory. Her books include: *Theories of Women's Studies* (1983), *Test-Tube Women* (1984), *Man-Made Women* (1985), *Infertility* (1989), *The Exploitation of a Desire* (1989), *Radical Voices* (1989), and *Angels of Power* (1991).

Janice G. Raymond is Professor of Women's Studies and Medical Ethics at the University of Massachusetts, Amherst, and Associate Director of the Institute on Women and Technology at MIT, Cambridge, USA. She has written extensively on the new reproductive technologies. Her most recent book is *Technological Injustice: Women and the New Reproductive Medicine* (1992).

Lynette J. Dumble is the Senior Research Fellow in the University of Melbourne's Department of Surgery at the Royal Melbourne Hospital and Visiting Professor of Surgery at the University of Texas, Houston, USA. She has published numerous articles in medical and scientific journals in the areas of transplantation, immuno-suppression (including prostaglandins), and medical ethics.

Spinifex Press is an independent feminist press, publishing innovative and controversial fiction and non-fiction by Australian and international authors. Direct mail orders by cheque or credit card are welcome. Books are available from 504 Queensberry Street, North Melbourne, Victoria 3051, Australia or from selected, good bookshops.

Spinifex is an Australian native desert grass that is drought resistant and holds the earth together. In central Australia spinifex grass is traditionally burnt by Aboriginal people as a means of regenerating the land.

RU 486
Misconceptions, Myths and Morals

by
Renate Klein
Janice G. Raymond
Lynette J. Dumble

SPINIFEX PRESS
Australia

AAY7612

Spinifex Press Pty Ltd,
504 Queensberry Street,
North Melbourne, Vic. 3051
Australia

First published by Spinifex Press, 1991
This is a co-publication of Spinifex Press, Melbourne, Australia and
The Institute on Women and Technology, MIT, Cambridge, USA.

Typeset in 11/12.4 pt New Baskerville by Claire Warren, Melbourne
Production by Sylvana Scannapiego, Island Graphics, Melbourne
Made and Printed in Australia by The Book Printer, Victoria
The contents of this book have been printed on 100% recycled paper

National Library of Australia
Cataloguing-in-Publication entry:
CIP
Klein, Renate.
 RU 486: misconceptions, myths and morals.

 Bibliography.
 ISBN 1 875559 01 9.

 1. Mifepristone. 2. Abortion. I. Raymond, Janice G.
 II. Dumble, Lynette J. (Lynette Joyce), 1946–   . III.
 Title.

363.46

ACKNOWLEDGEMENTS

We would like to extend special gratitude to those who helped in various ways with this project. For their thoughtful comments on the manuscript-in-progress, we thank Rita Arditti, Gena Corea, Susan Hawthorne, Amy Hines, H. Patricia Hynes, Judy Luce and Jocelynne Scutt. Renate Sadrozinski and Susanne von Paczensky clarified, in several discussions, the simplicity of suction abortion. Elfie Mayer provided documentation of the earlier anti-prostaglandin movement in Germany. The women at ISIS International in Geneva kindly searched their files for articles on both RU 486 and prostaglandin. Among those we interviewed, we thank Paul van Look for information on the WHO trials and Y. Q. Yang and J. T. Wu for discussing their research with us. Françoise Laborie sent us material from France and Hélène Rouch provided useful contacts in Paris. In Australia, Marie Iglesias and Christine Ewing helped with the typing of the references, Rose Mildenhall with library searches, and Pierre Smith with the translation of discs and preparation of transparencies. And without Chris Game's computer wizardry – not to mention her patience and invaluable donation of time – we would not have retained our sanity while persisting with three incompatible computer systems.

Because this report has been co-published in both Australia and the United States, we thank Claire Warren and Sylvana Scannapiego (Australia), and Jane Bradley and Karen Jones (USA) for their expertise and contributions in producing this work.

CONTENTS

CHAPTER FOUR

CONCLUSION   112

ENDNOTES

BIBLIOGRAPHY   132

INTRODUCTION

Initial euphoria greeted the arrival of RU 486, the new chemical abortifacient. Billed as a remarkable scientific achievement and miracle drug, plaudits and pundits hailed it as the 'magic bullet' of the decade.

In April 1991, however, the 'magic bullet' killed its first reported victim. The French Ministry of Health announced the first woman's death associated with RU 486. Officials stated that a thirty-one-year-old woman, in her 13th pregnancy, had died of cardiovascular complications resulting from the synthetic prostaglandin, Nalador (sulprostone), which is given in conjunction with RU 486 (thus we refer to the procedure hereafter as RU 486/PG). Significantly, the death occurred in France, the country which has performed over 60,000 chemical abortions and has the most experience with the drug.

The promotion of RU 486/PG is happening at an historical point when 50 million abortions per year are performed worldwide. Conventional abortion is a safe and effective procedure, yet 200,000 women – the majority from developing countries – die annually from illegal and botched terminations. The number of women who have died from poorly performed and clandestine abortions during the last ten years in Nicaragua, for example, is greater than the number of women who were killed by the contras during that same time period.

In the United States, there are over 1.5 million elective abortions annually. The number of women who die yearly from abortions in the United States is vastly lower than the abortion mortality figures of women in developing countries. US deaths have decreased from 2.3 per 100,000 abortions during the years 1972–78, to 0.8 deaths per 100,000 in 1979–85. Almost 98 per cent of all first trimester abortions in the United States are performed using curettage – mainly suction curettage. A large proportion of them do not require general anaesthesia (Atrash *et al.*, 1990: 58–69). Conventional abortion is one of the safest and easiest medical procedures, when done by trained and competent practitioners.

The introduction of RU 486/PG is taking place as anti-abortion fundamentalism is gaining ground. Since the Roe versus Wade Supreme Court decision in 1973 making abortion legal in the United States, anti-abortion forces have incrementally chipped away at the limited gains of this legal decision. Over the last 15 years, they have succeeded in depriving poor women of federal abortion funding and in challenging various provisions of the law, such as the necessity for parental consent to a minor's abortion. In 1989, the conservatively weighted US Supreme Court gave states the right to limit and regulate abortions within their own jurisdictions.

Anti-abortion groups were said to be responsible for Roussel Uclaf, the pharmaceutical company that developed RU 486, withdrawing distribution of the chemical abortifacient in France in 1988, one month after the Health Ministry had given it marketing approval. The French government allegedly intervened and ordered the company to resume distribution of the drug. Since then, anti-abortion groups have been active in fighting its release in other countries, even for non-abortive purposes. All feminist literature promoting the distribution of RU 486/PG in the

United States makes mention of the need for concerned citizens to combat this anti-abortion fascism.

Unfortunately, objections to RU 486/PG have largely come from anti-abortionists. They have used health and safety concerns about RU 486/PG to advance their own campaign against women's right to abortion. They have raised many of the critical issues regarding the drug in a way that has defined the parameters of the debate as 'us against them'. There is, however, an urgent need for more informed feminist discussion of RU 486/PG, but *not* on the terms of the anti-abortionists. This discussion has been muted by the proponents' accusation that any woman who raises objections to the drug is playing into the hands of the right wing. Presumably, the recognition that women have independent critical judgements has been one of the vital legacies of this wave of feminism. Women have the right to safe and effective abortions, but women also have the right to question whether RU 486/PG fulfills those claims.

This report challenges the uncritical promotion of RU 486/PG by women's groups. The US-based Reproductive Health Technologies Project has brought women's health groups' representatives from, for example, the National Women's Health Network and the Federation of Feminist Health Centers together with officers from the Population Crisis Committee, Planned Parenthood, and NARAL (National Abortion Rights Action League) to serve on an advisory board. A major aim of this project has been to promote education supporting and distribution of RU 486/PG in the United States.

The Feminist Majority has also launched a current major mission to 'alert the public to the medical benefits of RU 486.' Primarily, it has been responsible for amassing thousands of signatures in a petition drive designed to pressure Roussel Uclaf to license and/or distribute the drug in the United States. Their educational packet of articles, mailed to those requesting information on the

3

drug, depends wholly on studies and statements prepared by the drug researchers. Each article includes within its authorship at least one member or affiliate of the Roussel Uclaf team.

We share the sense of embattlement that many women feel, given the right-wing anti-abortion gains of the last decade. We also understand the need for feminist groups to make coalitions with other organizations. We do *not* understand why this embattlement has so quickly turned into accepting the claims for RU 486/PG; and why the need for coalitions has translated into joining with many population groups that have had a history of promoting dangerous and debilitating drugs, devices, and public policies for women (see Conclusion).

We believe there is a pressing need for independent feminist research, analysis, and discussion of RU 486/PG that does not accept uncritically the conclusions of the drug company's research. Much of the positive reaction to RU 486/PG has thus far been based on these studies. This report is a comprehensive review and analysis of hundreds of medical and scientific articles on RU 486/PG, a large percentage of which have a connection with Roussel Uclaf and which reiterate the Roussel Uclaf findings.

Dominant assumptions about RU 486/PG need to be fundamentally re-examined, such as the claims for privatizing the abortion environment, and the drug's portrayal as a 'private, woman-controlled, safe and effective' means of abortion. There appears to be an unquestioning acceptance that RU 486/PG de-medicalizes abortion, whereas the reality of RU 486/PG treatment is that it re-medicalizes, i.e. more thoroughly medicalizes, the abortion experience for women. RU 486/PG treatment is administered solely under strict medical supervision at specialized medical centres, requires three or four visits to a medical service, and can be used effectively only within 42–49 days after a woman's last menstrual period, that is approximately 14–21 days after her first *missed* period. Many women, especially teenagers, do not know or do not admit that they are pregnant within this brief time period.

All these factors prompt larger questions. Does RU 486/PG increase women's reproductive choices? Many groups have promoted RU 486/PG as expanded *choice* for women. Yet in this instance, what is championed as the right to choose, strongly resembles the right to consume. Women are encouraged to become consumers for new technologies and drugs — for more and more dangerous ones in the case of RU 486. The reproductive choices offered are the medical-technical-corporate options made available. The view of many seems to be that as long as women give consent and are informed about selective aspects of the drug, they should be free to take their own risks with drugs and technologies that have media support but that we know little about. We contend that given the media hype and the lack of independent research on RU 486/PG, most women taking the drug are not informed and consent is relatively meaningless.

In addition to abortion, proposed uses of RU 486 include treatment for breast cancer, meningioma (brain tumor), glaucoma, dilation of the cervix in labor, thus preventing the need for a caesarian section, and even the treatment of cancer of the prostate in men. To anyone familiar with the history of reproductive drugs and technologies used on women, such as diethylstilbestrol (DES) and estrogen (now hormonal) replacement therapy, these claims have an all-too-wondrous ring of promise subsequently turned peril. How many times have women been told that this or that drug will save us from ourselves?

The promotional coverage of RU 486 in the media has been designed to raise public expectations of the drug. Much of the press coverage — mainstream and feminist — has treated it as the revolutionary reproductive drug of the century. Moreover, the promise of research and treatment with RU 486/PG has capitalized on a common enemy of women's rights and scientific research. 'Both women's health care and freedom of research are being sacrificed by allowing anti-abortion extremists to block the production and distribution of RU 486' (The Feminist Majority Foundation Communiqué, 1990).

This report is a critical professional and feminist response to many issues raised by the research and development on RU 486/PG. We look first at the history of the drug — where it was tested and on whom; curious events in France that inspired Roussel Uclaf in 1988 to launch, then withdraw, and then return the drug to the market; and problems of marketing in the United States and other countries.

We examine, in turn, the complexion of the drug. What do they/we really know about the way it works in regard to not only the reproductive cycle but its impact on other parts of the body? What about the long-term effects of RU 486/PG on women's subsequent fertility? Since both drugs are known to cross the placenta, there is also some data that points to a teratogenic effect on the embryo after a failed chemical abortion. What are the contraindications for and complications of the drug? How are they represented in the medical literature?

We question why many serious side-effects have been downplayed, and the methods of minimizing their importance. Why is more and more pain, for example, represented as less and less of a problem for women? The minimizing of other complications such as post-treatment bleeding, which can be both long-lasting and severe, is another area of analysis. Some women have needed transfusions, and others have required conventional abortions after chemical abortions have failed.

Because RU 486 is administered with prostaglandins, its effect on the immune system must be studied further. When used in organ transplant procedures, much smaller doses of prostaglandins than are administered with RU 486 inhibit the immune response. Furthermore, prostaglandins have been used widely for years as an abortion method with painful and tragic consequences (see Chapter Four). The reluctance of the medical profession to publish these results has created an unawareness of just how dangerous prostaglandins are for women.

How have the comparisons between conventional and chemical abortions been treated? Comparisons have been framed as 'surgical versus chemical' abortion when, in reality, most conventional abortions do not and should not require surgery nor general anaesthesia. Also, what is the language that governs the representation of RU 486/PG to the public? Finally, what are the unasked and unanswered questions?

The interests, health, and safety of women cannot be served by relegating these issues to the background. As bad as the political climate may be in the United States and other countries surrounding women's right to abortion, we cannot allow that climate to dictate acceptance of a combination drug treatment that has not been investigated critically, and from a non-aligned perspective, i.e. a perspective not affiliated with the interests of the medical researchers, drug companies, and population control organizations. We also cannot allow the euphoria over RU 486/PG to decrease or eliminate conventional abortion centres and methods. If chemical abortions become the dominant treatment, and in future years the dangers are realized, women may well be faced with substantially reduced conventional abortion services.

Although it is claimed that RU 486 has been given to over 60,000 women in France, there is more about the drug that is unknown than known. It has been used extensively in only one country for a short period of time. It has been administered in France to a homogeneous population — white and middle class — a country in which surgical, not suction, abortion is the dominant alternative to chemical abortion. We know very little about its differential impact on women of color. Black women have a significantly higher incidence of fibroids, and Native American women have a higher incidence of diabetes than white women; and many women of minority status, as well as poor women, have a high rate of pre-existing anemia (Pearson in *Los Angeles Times*, 1990: E-14). For example, it has been estimated that 64 per cent of the women involved in a Bangladesh study had anemia, 25 per cent of which was severe. In India, the situation is worse (Le Grand, 1990: 21). All these factors have been cited as contraindications for the drug.

Little is known about the drug's both long- and short-term consequences. The conditions under which it is administered require careful scrutiny, particularly the sequential nature of the treatment and the need for close medical supervision. And most currently available prostaglandins must be kept refrigerated. These conditions have particular ramifications if RU 486/PG is to be distributed in developing countries or, for that matter, in areas of western countries where poor, Black, and other minority women do not have access to the kind of middle-class medical services and follow-up provided for French women undergoing chemical abortions. For these and other reasons, the 6th International Women and Health Meeting, held in the Philippines in November 1990, issued a resolution opposing the trials and the introduction of RU 486/PG especially in third world countries.

It is these unknowns, these background issues, these minimalized areas, that this report investigates in depth.

CHAPTER ONE

The History of RU 486

RU 486 is a recent discovery. In April 1980, Georges Teutsch and Daniel Philibert of Roussel Uclaf, with French scientist Etienne-Emile Baulieu, a consultant to the company, succeeded in synthesizing RU 486, a steroid now with the trade name Miféngyne (mifepristone).[1] Ten years later, Roussel Uclaf employees Ulmann, Teutsch and Philibert denied that the research which led to the synthesis of RU 38486 (later shortened to RU 486) was performed with the intention of discovering an abortifacient. They claimed it was a by-product of the company's active search for a molecule which would bind strongly with the *glucocorticoid receptor*. However, 'Initial tests in several species soon revealed that RU 486 was [also] a *progesterone* antagonist' (Ulmann *et al.*, 1990: 45 [our emphasis]). Baulieu's long-standing interest in hormonal contraception prompted Roussel Uclaf to focus further investigation of RU 486 on the drug's potential to impede ovulation, act as a 'morning-after' pill, and interrupt pregnancy.

A mere 17 months of animal research on rabbits, rats and monkeys was deemed sufficient to judge RU 486 promising and 'safe' enough to warrant clinical trials on women. As early as October 1981, the first study on eleven women took place at the University Hospital in Geneva,

Switzerland (Herrmann *et al.*, 1982). Promoters of RU 486 such as Sheldon Segal, director for population sciences at the Rockefeller Foundation, admitted this move to be 'an unusual example of the rapid clinical application of basic research findings...' (1990: 691). A member of the Geneva team indicated that the rush to clinical trials was a move to 'beat' other pharmaceutical companies researching a similar compound (Rina Nissim, pers. comm. to RK, June 1990).[2] Indeed the competition came from the US-owned company Sterling Winthrop (epostane), and the German company Schering Laboratories (two ZK analogues, onapristone and lilopristone). Currently, neither drug is marketed for abortion purposes.

In the Geneva trial, eleven women, six to eight weeks pregnant, received 200 mg of RU 486 per day for three consecutive days. Nine pregnancies were terminated, in eight women after five days, in one woman after nine days. One of the women initially claimed as 'success' later needed a uterine evacuation and, in another, heavy bleeding necessitated blood transfusion and emergency surgery (Baulieu, 1989a: 1811). The Paris newspaper *Libération* commented that, given these associated complications and risks, RU 486 was no 'abortion miracle'. *Libération* also reported that RU 486 is not only an anti-progesterone but an *anti-glucocorticosteroid* which can take the place of cortisone in the adrenal glands, and that contraindications emanating from this double action of the drug could be a problem (Lépiney, 1982: 2). This suspicion was confirmed in the first RU 486 toxicological study in monkeys, which led to adverse reactions affecting the adrenal glands (see Chapter Three for details).

Despite scant research on animals and the dubious results from Geneva, clinical trials on women began in France, Sweden, Australia, Holland, USA, England, Finland and China. Roussel Uclaf supplied the drug and its staff and consultants are listed among the authors of the resulting publications from many of these trials. André

Ulmann of Roussel Uclaf is even credited with designing a Chinese study of RU 486 (Zheng,1989).

In these trials, reported 'success rates' – that is the numbers of women for whom the administration of RU 486 resulted in a *complete* termination of their pregnancy without the need for further medical intervention – varied considerably from 54 per cent (Herrmann *et al.*, 1982), 60 per cent (Kovacs *et al.*, 1984) to 85 per cent (Couzinet *et al.*, 1986) and even 90 per cent (Grimes *et al.*, 1988). The research papers concluded that RU 486 was a promising alternative to conventional abortion, and a medical 'breakthrough', but the number of complete terminations achieved with this drug was well below the established 99 per cent of conventional abortion (Chavkin and Rosenfield, 1990). In order to improve these negative results, the next step in the development of the 'abortion pill' was to combine RU 486 with *prostaglandins*.

Since 1970 prostaglandins, which induce uterine contractions, have been used to initiate labor and to interrupt pregnancies throughout the world. The initial optimism about the use of prostaglandins for abortion was soon dampened by disappointing success rates and serious adverse effects. For these reasons, the European Women's Health Movement organized against the use of prostaglandins in the late 70s (see Chapter Four for details).

In spite of these known problems, Marc Bygdeman and Marja Liisa Swahn of the Karolinska Institute in Stockholm commenced the administration of RU 486 in combination with a prostaglandin (PG) following the earlier research of Csapo (see Chapter Four). Under the sponsorship of WHO in 1984, their small study included 34 women and seemed promising: complete abortions occurred in 32 women (94 per cent), (Bygdeman and Swahn, 1985). As a result of this research, RU486/PG was rapidly deemed superior to RU 486 alone. The majority of later studies[3] used varying doses of RU 486 in combination with different types of PGs which were administered as intramuscular

11

injections, suppositories or, as first reported in 1990, orally (Swahn *et al.*).[4] It is crucial to note that these clinical trials were undertaken without basic research into potential adverse effects from the *interaction* of the two drugs (see Chapter Four for further details).

Until the publication of the results of Chinese trials with RU 486/PG in 1989, which reported that 2321 women had participated in four multicenter clinical trials,[5] the numbers of women in the clinical trials were small. From the initial 11 women in the Geneva study, the numbers ranged from 35 (Vervest and Haspels, 1985) to 100 (Couzinet *et al.*, 1986) and 271 women (Grimes *et al.*, 1990). Grimes' figures were a total of all the women who had been administered the drug from 1984 to 1989 in his US trials). Even a 1989 WHO publication of a multicenter trial with eight medical centers participating included only 261 women. Two publications in 1990 reported larger numbers: Louise Silvestre of Roussel Uclaf and colleagues Dubois, Baulieu and Ulmann listed 2040 French women as participants in their study, and a UK multicentre trial had 588 participants, a number still significantly lower that the 50,000 to 60,000 women who are said to have undergone chemical abortion by the beginning of 1991.[6] Importantly, the three largest studies conducted to this point were either undertaken by Roussel Uclaf or were affiliated with the French company. As the authors of the UK multitrial paper acknowledged, they 'prepared their report from data provided by Roussel Uclaf' (UK Multicentre Trial, 1990: 480).[7] The general tenor in these publications is one of assured optimism. As Louise Silvestre and colleagues put it, 'We conclude that the administration of mifepristone [RU 486] followed by a small dose of a prostaglandin analogue is an effective and safe method for the early termination of pregnancy' (1990: 645).

Events in France

The history of RU 486 took a dramatic turn in 1988. In September, Roussel Uclaf was licensed by the French Ministry of Health to market RU 486. But on 26 October, Chairman Sakiz of Roussel suspended the distribution of RU 498. The press claimed that Sakiz' action was due to anti-abortionist threats to the company and its employees.[8] In an interview with the *New York Times* on 28 October, Etienne Baulieu commented, 'He [Sakiz] told me he hopes there is pressure to counteract the decision' (Simons, 1988: A1). Conveniently, the World Congress of Gynecology and Obstetrics in Rio de Janeiro, Brazil, was meeting at this very moment and included a Symposium on RU486 – organized by Baulieu, Segal and Roussel Uclaf – which sent a petition of 2000 names to Roussel Uclaf, protesting the withdrawal of the drug.

On 28 October 1988, the media reported that the French Minister of Health, Claude Evin, had ordered Roussel Uclaf to put RU 486 back on the market. (The French state owns 36.25 per cent of Roussel Uclaf which, however, is short of the 51 per cent required to enforce a decision.) Evin was quoted as saying that RU 486 had become 'moralement la proprieté des femmes' (Nau and Nouchi, 1988: 9). Since then, the slogan that RU 486 is 'the moral property of women', has been the battlecry of promoters of the drug, including some feminist groups in the USA, Australia and Switzerland. In France, RU 486 was officially back – under tight security – at hospitals and centers licensed to perform abortion in February 1989.

Two years later, in January 1991, a bizarre twist was added to the 'official' story. The French Government Council (Conseil d'Etat) reprimanded Health Minister Claude Evin for exceeding his power in ordering Roussel Uclaf to return RU 486 to the market in October 1988. Surprisingly, however, Evin now claims that he had *not* issued such an order because 'discussions and exchange of arguments with representatives from Roussel Uclaf had made recourse to this procedure unnecessary' (Vigy, 1991: 18). Combined with the exceedingly convenient timing of events from the Rio de Janeiro convention, this indicates a contrived history of events operative at all levels.

International Affirmation and Criticism

The decision to put RU 486 back on the market pertained only to France. Roussel Uclaf had decided not to market the drug in other countries.[9] Meanwhile, in November 1988, the US-based Reproductive Health Technologies Project was set up by the private consulting firm Bass and Howes in Washington. Assembling an unusual group of people (see Introduction), the Reproductive Technologies Health Project initiated a well-funded campaign which extends even to Australia. Here, its uncritical pro-RU 486 information packet has been distributed to all women's centers and state-based women's units. With the slogan 'New Technologies/New Choices' it began a campaign to convince politicians and the community at large to put pressure on Roussel Uclaf to distribute the drug in the USA and other countries.

The Reproductive Health Technologies Project is explicit in its support for the abortion pill – based on Roussel Uclaf material. Its packet contains a sample letter which should be sent to Roussel Uclaf and Hoechst to urge them to stop keeping American women – and women elsewhere in the world – from access to their 'moral property'. Their efforts were soon augmented by a 'historical campaign' from the Feminist Majority: 'RU 486 is safe and amazingly effective...it is simple', and, 'frankly, there are few steps as significant – and long-lasting – as the action we can take to bring RU 486 into the United States' (Communiqué, 1990). Moreover, both groups assert that RU 486 has enormous potential to treat other diseases from glaucoma to breast cancer. Both campaigns are also unequivocal in their assessment that the debate is entirely between the 'bad' anti-abortionists and the 'good' scientists who developed this miracle drug in the service of women. In August 1990, President Eleanor Smeal of the Feminist Majority visited the Paris headquarters of Roussel Uclaf and deposited 400 kg of signed petitions.

Support for RU 486 in the USA also came from the American Medical Assocation (Lee, 1990: 1). Louise Tyrer, vice president of medical affairs for National Planned Parenthood welcomed the decision 'for advancing a major scientific breakthrough such as RU 486' (*idem.*).

Others have speculated that it may be necessary to create a company that would solely test and market the drug. Such a possibility was also mentioned by David Grimes. He pointed out that 'RU 486 is a relatively simple molecule to synthesize' and that there were already half a dozen small Californian companies 'that want to run with this thing' and have requested his help. As Grimes put it, 'The big boys won't touch it' adding, 'The problem is that [to duplicate or import RU 486] you need the consent of Roussel Uclaf' (Krier, 1990: E 12).

Whether the idea of a special purpose company is a realistic possibility for introducing RU 486 into the USA remains to be seen. Peter Huber, Senior Fellow at the Manhattan Institute for Policy Research is sceptical. He commented that 'readying RU 486 for FDA approval could cost US$50 million to US$100 million in clinical tests and legal fees. . .as much as US$125 million to US$200 million into marketing and distribution costs' (Chapman, 1989: 13). In addition, there is the fear of litigation, as Huber puts it: the two to four per cent 'natural' birth defects in children might be blamed on RU 486.

In addition to Roussel Uclaf's reluctance to market RU 486 in the United States, there is the problem of the *prostaglandin* needed for combination treatment with RU 486. Despite FDA approval for PGs in other areas, for example approval of Cytotec (misoprostol) as an anti-ulcer drug, (see Chapter Four), no PG is approved for abortion purposes in the US.

The situation is different in the UK where Roussel Uclaf applied to the Ministry of Health for a marketing license, approval for which, according to Tony Seaton of Roussel Uclaf UK, 'could take from 18 months to two years' (pers. comm. to RK, 28 July 1990). In early 1991, it was rumored that the licensing procedure had been speeded up and approval would be granted by the end of January. Approval was finally granted on 3 July 1991. No application for marketing approval has been made in Australia. In August 1990, former Federal Minister Margaret Reynolds urged women to undertake a letter writing campaign to put pressure on Roussel Uclaf (Gillies, 1990). Another action undertaken to bolster chemical abortion came in November 1990 at a conference sponsored by the Abortion Providers Federation of Australasia in Melbourne. Etienne Baulieu was the invited keynote speaker and with the exception of the critical voice of one of us (LD) all speakers hailed RU 486 as a major medical breakthrough which was being unfairly withheld from Australian women. However, a spokesperson from Roussel Uclaf–Australia (Sydney) repeated that they had not yet submitted an application to the Federal Department of Health. Similarly with New Zealand, Roussel Uclaf said they were not open to invitation (Coney, 1990a: 11).

Predictably, Australian anti-abortion groups protested promotion of RU 486/PG. 'This drug kills unborn babies' said Margaret Tighe, Chairman [*sic*] of Right to Life Australia. 'There are complications with the drug and they are frightened they might face litigation' (Gillies, 1990).[10] Outside the right-wing perspective, the only criticism of chemical abortion was heard on TV and radio in Australia and New Zealand where our non-aligned feminist perspective opened the debate.[11]

In 1989, RU 486 made the news again in France when, in order to recoup its investment costs, Roussel Uclaf set the price of RU 486 at FF517 (approx. US$100). This was at odds with the Ministry of Health's decision that had fixed the drug's price at FF93.5 (approx. US$17) (Coles, 1989: 6). The result appears to be a compromise in favor of Roussel: *La Révue Prescrire* of July/August 1990 (p. 286) quotes FF265 (approx. US$48) for 600 mg Mifégyne (three pills), noting that the cost for the *initial* consultation including prescription of RU 486 is FF388 (US$70), and the *total* cost for chemical abortion is set at FF1408 (approx. US$255).[12] In comparison, surgical abortion in France costs $150 (*ISIS Women's Health Journal*, 1990: 8).

An even greater controversy erupted in early 1990, when an international group of scientists and doctors based at the Necker Hospital in Paris, reviewed the data of 30,000 women who had used RU 486 (Ewing, 1990: 1) and issued a stern warning against it. They urged the Ministry of Health 'to enforce what was inevitable: the immediate suppression of the distribution and use of RU 486' because of 'the grave secondary effects of chemical abortion which is falsely seen as an alternative to surgical abortion' (Kami, 1990: 9). Their concern arose from the associated bleeding necessitating emergency curettage and sometimes blood transfusion, from reduced hemoglobin and hemocrit levels, and from two severe cases of cardiovascular accidents associated with the addition of prostaglandin to RU 486 (see Chapter Four).[13] Shortly afterwards, 15 centers which performed chemical abortion responded by defending RU 486/PG abortion (Caro, 1990: 10). Nevertheless, the 'Direction de la Pharmacie et du Médicament' (DMPH, the French equivalent of the US FDA or Australian Drug Evaluation Branch) had already demanded that Roussel Uclaf issue stricter guidelines. On 20 April 1990, the company sent a circular to all clinics providing chemical abortion. Roussel Uclaf specified that cardiovascular risk factors, e.g. heavy smoking, obesity, elevated serum lipid (related to cholesterol), diabetes and high blood pressure restrict the use of chemical abortion. They also cautioned against administering it to women over 35 (see Chapter Two).

The Role of the International Press

What has the role of the press internationally been in the RU 486 debate? It is fair to say that the controversies in France over the safety of the two drugs were not reported. The only exceptions were articles in *Le Monde* and *Le Quotidien du Médecin* where some of the curious events in France were described. *Le Monde* reported that the reason prompting Roussel Uclaf to withdraw the drug initially in France came from concerns that were voiced about complications (Nouchi, 1988: 12).

The overwhelming majority of articles in the USA, England and Australia portray the controversy over RU 486/PG as a simplistic battle between pro- and anti-abortion forces. Newspaper and magazine articles hail chemical abortion as 'safe and painless' and uncritically repeat medical claims of 'the drug's reduced rate of complication over surgical abortion' (Simons, 1988: A1). Further, conventional abortion is reported as always traumatic and dangerous because it is 'surgery' which necessitates general anaesthesia (thereby denying the existence of suction curettage with a local anaesthethic; see Chapter Two). Chemical abortion is presented as superior: 'The pill [RU 486] minimises the risk that surgery carries' (Sapsted, 1991: 40–42). The press has also failed to understand that chemical abortion does *not* lead to de-medicalization but rather to re-medicalization, i.e. to a more thorough medicalization of pregnancy termination (see Chapter Two). Other press reports repeat Baulieu's claims that it is our moral duty to make RU 486/PG available in the third world. 'Denying this pill to women is basically signing the death warrant for the 200,000 women who die [worldwide] annually from abortion' (Tyer quoted in Chapman, 1989: 13). José Barzelatto, former WHO director concurs and adds that, 'for the first time in medical history, we have a safe, effective and acceptable medical method of terminating pregnancy' (Kingman, 1989: 4). This ignores the fact that many women die because abortion is *illegal* in many developing countries and that the availability of chemical abortion would not change this. Of the few critical articles, two came from New Zealand in which feminist health critic and author Sandra Coney drew attention to Baulieu's inaccurate reporting of complications from his own study (Coney, 1990a and b).[14]

The feminist press internationally – as well as feminist health groups in general – have predominantly reacted to the news of RU 486 with optimism, if not enthusiasm. In 1990, the German feminist magazine *Emma* ran two articles, both urging women to put pressure on Roussel Uclaf and Hoechst to make the drug available outside France (Rauch 1990: 6; zur Nieden 1990: 26–27). In 1988 and 1989, the Women's Global Network on Reproductive Rights repeatedly published articles in their *Newsletter* assuming a similar position of support for RU 486 as the Feminist Majority and the Reproductive Health Technologies Project in the USA. *Newsletter* editor, Marge Berer, for instance, reported from a workshop on RU 486 at a 1989 British conference where she was joined by David Baird, a member of the British Multicentre Trial team, André Ulmann from Roussel Uclaf, and Rebecca Cook, a member of the US Reproductive Health Technologies Project. Berer concluded that she left the conference convinced that the women's health movement must join the international campaign to make RU 486 available, especially in the third world (Berer, 1989: 3). In the same issue, Janet Callum and Carol Downer from the US Federation of Feminist Health Centers enthusiastically describe their visit to a French hospital where RU 486 was administered and to Roussel Uclaf where they talked with André Ulmann.

Only a few feminist publications carried reports on the pill that were accompanied by cautionary remarks. An article in the German periodical *Clio* (republished and translated in *Connexions*, 1989: 15) noted that RU 486 has not proven harmless and reminded their readers of earlier 'miracle drugs' such as DES and Duogynon (one of the early heavy-dose contraceptive pills). They also said, 'the introduction of chemicals to the body can be no less intrusive than surgery' (p. 15) and pointed out that RU 486 causes greater blood loss than conventional termination, thus reinforcing medical supervision. Finally, they cautioned against 'fooling ourselves with false hopes that this new pill might expand abortion options in countries which thus far prohibited abortions'. Similarly, Marie Vallée of the Quebec Family Planning Federation, in an article entitled 'RU 486 – Another Fake Miracle?' wrote in 1989 that nothing is known about long-term effects, future fertility and babies born after repeated use of the abortion pill. Valleé cautioned against rushing to support this drug and asked whether it is really the much-awaited solution to women's 20-year demand 'for more research into products that do not endanger their health and the health of their children' (*ISIS Women's Health Journal* 1989: 32).

In response to the *WGNRR Newsletter* articles in favor of RU 486, Rina Nissim, long-term women's health activist and author, expressed disagreement with Callum, Downer and Berer (1989: 5):

> I'm surprised to find no criticism, doubts or disadavantages of RU 486 described in those two articles ... Since when do we feminists trust a multinational pharmaceutical company like this, without taking the time to search for information about possible short-term and long-term side effects, risk for the woman etc? Is Roussel Uclaf the most reliable source for this information? Did you forget what counter-information is about?

Nissim then described events that took place in Geneva in 1982, with regard to the first trial. Working with the Dispensaire des Femmes at that time, she had close contacts with Rolf Wyss, a member of the clinical trial team at the University Hospital who expressed considerable reservation about RU 486 (pers. comm. to RK, June 1990).[15]

Nissim also reinforced the *Le Monde* article suggesting that the withdrawal of RU 486 in France in 1988, might not only have been because of the anti-abortionists, but because of complications from the pill:

> It was strategically very smart, because they [Roussel Uclaf] were requested to bring it back. Women today have the impression that they are getting something others wanted to refuse them, so they are more likely to accept or be silent about the disadvantages.[16]

In June 1990, the Dutch-based group, WEMOS Women and Pharmaceuticals, organized a seminar on RU 486, with speakers from the Dutch Abortion Providers, the WHO and a French Hospital which administers the drug and WEMOS. In spite of the optimistic promotion of RU 486/PG-abortion by Bernard Maria, French abortion provider and co-author of some Roussel Uclaf studies, serious concerns were raised regarding the drug's safety and efficacy. Specifically, seminar participants queried third-world applications; it was feared a black market might be established with disastrous consequences. WHO representative Paul van Look also pointed out that because of RU 486's anti-glucocorticoid activity, a more 'pure' antiprogestin might be developed in time. The seminar ended on a cautionary note: 'Given the knowledge of the abortion pill at the moment, it doesn't seem wise to promote it on a large scale' (*WEMOS Proceedings,* 1990: 36).

The 'Father' of the Abortion Pill?

The future of RU486/PG abortion remains unresolved. In a 1990 interview with the *New York Times,* Etienne Baulieu had accused both Roussel Uclaf and WHO of being slow to distribute the drug, especially in third world countries. Commenting on Hirochi Nagashima, the head of WHO's reproduction unit, Baulieu said, 'The man says he's afraid that American money will be cut off if an RU 486 program comes under the WHO umbrella' (Riding, July 29: 15). Baulieu felt strongly that this impasse must be ended, and that because of 'its simplicity...RU 486 could have a dramatic effect in reducing the number of illegal abortions and related maternal deaths and injuries throughout the third world.' As he put it: 'How can we ignore that 500 women die every day as a result of badly executed abortions?' Distancing himself from Baulieu's accusations, Roussel Uclaf's Chairman Sakiz responded that marketing in the third world 'would be the quickest way to sabotage the product'. Following from discussions with Chinese and Indian health authorities Sakiz said, 'they told me it would be impossible to control a product of that kind in their countries' (Nau, 1990 August 19: 16).

During his mission to Australia and New Zealand in November 1990, Etienne Baulieu refused to discuss problems with the drug. Asked about possible malformations in the babies of women who continue pregnancies after the failure of RU 486, he said: 'You have to take my word.' When asked about administration of RU 486/PG in the so-called developing world, he commented that the situation was so bad anyway that the pill would be an improvement:

> Don't tell me it would be perfect. Nothing is perfect including particularly in developing countries in terms of health and women's health. But if, for the reason [*sic*] I've said, no anaesthesia, no infection, no perforations, it will be a progress. *We'll see a few catastrophes.* But remember we will probably reduce the death toll by I don't know, 90 per cent or something, because all these horrible complications will be wiped out by the use of a medical technique. (Newztel Log, Radio New Zealand: 8, emphasis ours).[17]

The risk of 'a few catastrophes' became real when the French pharmacovigilance network alerted the Ministry of Health to the death of a woman from chemical abortion.

On 8 April 1991, the Ministry of Health issued a *Communiqué* stating that a 31-year-old woman had died from cardio-vascular shock (heart failure) shortly after an injection of the prostaglandin Nalador (sulprostone) in conjunction with Myfégyne (RU 486). The first of 'a few catastrophes' had taken place, *not* in the third world but in high-tech France, where the safety requirements in case of emer-gency (e.g. equipment, medications) should have been met. Few details were released, but the *Communiqué* did point out that the young woman was a heavy smoker and in her 13th pregnancy (other sources mentioned that she was the mother of 11 children), and that in 1990, the Ministry of Health had warned against the use of RU 486/PG by smokers. Roussel Uclaf also revealed that the prostaglandin Nalador used independent of RU 486 was implicated in the deaths of three other women and four additional women who had suffered non-fatal heart attacks (quoted in Riding, 1991).

The company's response to the RU 486/Nalador death was simple: switch to another prostaglandin – gemeprost – which, although administered as a vaginal suppository requires increasing the dosage significantly from 0.25 mg to 1 mg (*idem.*, see also Chapter Four). On 19 April, the Health Ministry ruled that RU 486/PG was not to be administered to women who have smoked for more than two years or are older than 35. Further, it had decided to reduce the dosage of Nalador to 0.125 mg or alternatively to use 1 mg of Cervagem (gemeprost), and also mentioned that oral prostaglandin administration was under investi-gation.

Rather than expressing distress and bewilderment over the woman's death, Baulieu on the *same* day announced his latest experiments with women using an oral prostaglandin. As he put it, the oral prostaglandin was 'simpler, . . . less painful and possibly safer' than his previous promise for safe and effective abortion (Altman, 1991: C3; but see also Chapter Four for adverse effects of misoprostol).[18] When asked in a telephone interview when he first became aware of the dangers of Nalador (sulprostone) on Radio National, Australia, Baulieu's reply was, 'about three weeks ago' (Delaney, 22 April 1991)!

CHAPTER TWO

Claims for RU 486/PG Abortion

Privacy versus Control

Many of the claims about RU 486 are based on its supposed privatization of the abortion experience. Ellen Goodman, for example, in her syndicated column, calls for the marketing of RU 486 in the United States. 'What could be more private than taking a pill? How could a state control swallowing?' (1989: 11). Like Goodman, the media presentation of the new abortion pill in western countries tends to simplify and idealize the drug. The going wisdom holds that a woman pops a pill in the privacy of her own home and the pregnancy disappears.

The medical literature tells another story, belying the myth of the do-it-yourself abortion. Yet here too, the *rhetoric* of more control for women over the abortion experience co-exists with an entirely different *reality*. At a European meeting of gynecologists and obstetricians in 1987, Etienne Baulieu proclaimed that '. . . RU 486 could be a prototype of the second generation of ways of giving women more control of their fertility' (Baulieu, 1988b: 128). But in the same medical journal article, on the same page, and in the same paragraph, he also said: ' . . . it should be given under strict medical supervision in specialized centers' (*idem.*). So what are women to make of these conflicting claims and this effective doublespeak?

The clearest answer lies in the medical journal articles themselves. The conclusions that much of the medical literature draws are not consistent with the findings that the articles present. Additionally, every article, without exception, remarks that RU 486 should be administered only under strict medical supervision. The *reality* of medical surveillance is not simply physician oversight from a distance, but a highly medicalized, multi-step, time-consuming procedure which, for many women, involves continuous suffering and pain. This treatment regimen deserves careful scrutiny.

1. A woman seeking a chemical abortion must submit to a physical examination and pregnancy test. This includes a pelvic examination to see if there is any uterine bleeding or previous pelvic infection. During the physical examination, women should be checked for contra-indications, making the drug more dangerous for certain women. Most centers, now testing or administering the new abortion pill, use vaginal ultrasonography, i.e., sound waves that project a picture of the embryo on a screen to estimate gestational age of the pregnancy; and/or a determination of serum human chorionic gonadotropin (β-hCG) to confirm and define the age of a woman's pregnancy.

2. Depending on the legal situation in a particular country, many centers impose a waiting period of at least 24 hours or more after which a woman must return to the clinic or hospital for RU 486, given in tablet form (usually three). Contrary to the popular picture of the pill-popping abortion, a woman does not take these tablets home but usually swallows them in the presence of a nurse or doctor while she is at the clinic. This has been one of the myths supporting the privatization argument for RU 486. Some feminists have claimed that women eventually will be able to obtain RU 486/PG at the local supermarket. However, a woman *must* go to a

clinic or other medical center to obtain the tablets and return to the center for several visits. During the 48 hours between RU 486 and PG administration, women are required not to smoke or drink alcohol.

3. Procedures at this point vary. Some centers that give RU 486 alone require the woman to visit the clinic seven days after RU 486 administration to confirm that the embryo has been expelled completely. Most centers, however, now administer prostaglandins in concert with RU 486 to hasten and strengthen the contractions that will ultimately propel the embryo from the uterus. Thus women once again must return to the clinic for a prostaglandin injection, vaginal prostaglandin suppositories or, more recently, oral prostaglandins. The prostaglandins are usually given 36–48 hours after RU 486 administration because it takes this time to fully sensitize the myometrium (part of the uterine lining) to contract (see Chapter Four for an alternative theory). When the woman returns to the medical center for the prostaglandins, she is given another pelvic examination, the second one in 48 hours. Since the two cardiovascular accidents, which occurred in France after the administration of prostaglandins, women are now required to lie prone and have their blood pressure measured every half hour during and after PG administration. Again, this warrants further medical supervision, restricted to a medical center equipped with an electrocardiogram, cardiorespirator, and coronary spasm medication (*La Révue Prescrire*, 1990: 288).

4. Then the wait begins. Many clinics keep women prone for three to four hours, in the hope that the embryo will be expelled before sending them home. Other women wait longer hours, days, and some even weeks. The only thing private about RU 486 is that the final stage of the abortion, the expulsion of the embryo, often happens at home – or someplace else. To call this an at-home abortion is deceptive, to say the least, since most of the

treatment transpires in the clinic or hospital and is extremely medicalized. What actually happens at home can be an excruciatingly long wait for the embryo to be expelled from the uterus, accompanied by pain, bleeding, vomiting, nausea, and other complications that are drawn out over a substantially lengthy period of time, compared with a conventional abortion.

5. Finally, a woman must return several days later for a physician's examination to make sure abortion is complete. (Some studies mention as many as three follow–up appointments, e.g. Hill *et al.*, 1990a: 415). Again, vaginal ultrasound and/or a determination of ß-hCG is used to ascertain whether the pregnancy has been terminated and whether the embryonic tissue has been totally expelled. At this point the woman receives another pelvic examination, the third within a time period of usually eight days. The pelvic examination, vaginal ultrasound, and other instruments used internally in chemical abortion are important to emphasize, because women have been led to believe that an RU 486/PG abortion is free of medical instruments inserted into the body. This misrepresent-ation singles out only suction curettage as an invasive internal or instrumental procedure. In actual fact, chemical abortion involves the use of more interventionist instrumentation than conventional abortion.

6. If abortion is not complete, then a conventional abortion is performed. Between two and 13.4 per cent of women undergoing RU 486/PG terminations endure double abortion jeopardy (Gao *et al.*, 1988).

How does the claim that RU 486 is a private means of abortion square with the claim that it needs close medical supervision? It doesn't. Physicians have been very explicit that RU 486 will never be available over the counter for do-it-yourself abortions. Allan Templeton, professor of obstet-rics and gynecology at the University of Aberdeen, who is leading the British trials admits that, 'To maintain safety you require extremely close medical supervision' (*Sunday Times*, 30 October 1988).

How, then, are women presumed to control this new abortion method? What is the privacy and de-medicalization that has been so touted in the promotional literature? Privacy and control by what/whose standards? In the minds of many, both privacy and control seem to be equated with any method that is non-conventional. In reality, the RU 486/PG abortion method increases, rather than decreases, the lack of privacy and the lack of women's control over the abortion experience. The only thing different about an RU 486/PG abortion is the *rhetoric* of control which hardly matches the *reality* of strict and prolonged medical supervision. Measured by the number of doctor's visits, and the duration of time from visit one to visit three, or four (at which point the woman is back to square one of conventional abortion), we are talking about a non-private, extensively medicalized, and complicated abortion method.

Additionally, the anonymity of a woman's abortion is precluded by registration. Under French law, the abortion pill's use is tightly controlled. It is administered solely at designated family planning centers – the only place any type of abortion can be performed there – and is not available from individual doctors or pharmacies. In England, the next country where RU 486/PG is to be distributed and marketed, the 1967 Abortion Act requires that abortion technology and drugs be given exclusively in hospitals and clinics licensed under the act. Furthermore, all the trials have been closely controlled as in France, not simply because they are trials but, as many of the researchers and clinicians readily admit, because RU 486/PG is not safe enough to administer without close medical supervision. What happens, now, to Ellen Goodman's original question: 'How could a state control swallowing?' Easily, when a country, even for the best of reasons, controls the procedure in the way that France, England, and others currently do.

Likewise, the Fund for Feminist Majority, which has conducted an international campaign to bring RU 486/PG to the United States, claims that the pill would divest anti-abortion groups of 'one of their most effective tactics – open harassment and violence at abortion clinics. Because RU 486 can be administered at any doctor's office – not just at abortion clinics – picketing becomes meaningless!' (The Feminist Majority Foundation *Communiqué*, 1990). RU 486/PG has also been represented in the feminist press as being available from 'the local pharmacy' and thereby 'technologically bypassing' the anti-abortion movement. This claim is blatantly misleading since nowhere is RU 486 administered at 'any doctor's office.' Nor do hospitals and other medical services simply dispense RU 486/PG. It is only administered as a multi-step, *on-the-premise* procedure. These medical services, among them many clinics, can be picketed just as easily as the present conventional abortion clinics. Tony Seaton of Roussel Uclaf UK deplores that the general public incorrectly believes that RU 486 will be available from GPs. He reconfirmed that every pill will be numbered to ensure the strictest possible control and total restriction to licensed abortion clinics (pers. comm. to RK, 26 June 1991).

Doctors assert that the abortion pill will not be available at the pharmacy because it requires strict medical supervision, at the same time that they proclaim that RU 486/PG is a safe, streamlined, and privatized means of abortion for women. In an interview in the *Los Angeles Times*, David Grimes admitted that although he believes, 'We've got to get doctors and medical people out of the process,' he likes the stringent controls that now surround the drug (Grimes, quoted in Krier, 1990: E–12). But many feminists seem to believe that women will control the drug, and that the RU 486 abortion experience relieves women of the burdens of interventionist medicine and anti-abortion harassment. There appears to be an immense disparity in definitions of self-administration, privacy, and women's control of the abortion procedure when defined by the medical researchers and clinicians, and when defined by everyday people.

Safety versus Contraindications/Complications

There are a host of conditions, contraindications, and complications that expose the fallacy of the 'safe and effective' claims for RU 486/PG abortion. To begin, close medical supervision is necessary to establish the existence and length of pregnancy; to monitor bleeding and possibly perform a blood transfusion; to administer narcotic analgesics if women experience severe pain; to use ultrasound to determine complete expulsion of the embryo and tissue after the final treatment protocol; and to perform a conventional abortion if the chemical abortion is incomplete and/or the pregnancy continues. Added to this fact is that many women worldwide do not seek – or have access to – medical treatment promptly enough for chemical abortion to work. Particularly in developing countries women may not be able to obtain timely treatment, or the immense surveillance protocol now established as routine for chemical abortions. They must travel to a medical center several times – usually from a distance – for the various steps of treatment and testing. The problems of access and monitoring are equally real for many poor, indigenous, rural and other minority women in industrialized countries as well as the obvious difficulties for women in non-industrialized countries, who have no opportunity to receive this multi-step medical backup that is essential for minimum RU 486/PG abortion safety.

Those who have administered RU 486/PG report compliance and follow-up problems in the white, middle-class, western world. When asked whether there was any succeeding supervision to ascertain the future fertility of women who underwent RU 486/PG abortions in the Southern California trials, Daniel Mishell responded: '. . . we cannot even get the patients to return to have their blood drawn' (Mishell, quoted in Grimes *et al.*, 1988: 1311). Likewise, there have been difficulties in getting women to return for sequential treatments of RU 486 and prostaglandins, as well as final tests to determine complete termination of pregnancy (Silvestre *et al.*, 1990: 646). Additionally, a study done by Hill *et al.* mentions that seven per cent of women did not return for a seven day follow-up appointment, 15 per cent did not return for a 14 day follow-up appointment, and 13 per cent did not return for a final 28 day appointment (1990a: 415). Any medical treatment involving multiple steps is fraught with non-compliance. This is particularly true for abortion where the added moral, legal, and physical barriers make it more difficult for women to obtain even a one-step abortion procedure.

A nurse who was part of the US trials undertaken by David Grimes in Southern California relates – in a letter to the *Los Angeles Times* – that she was one of the non-success stories of the US abortion pill experiment. After 12 hours of severe cramping and vomiting, she went to the County university hospital emergency room where she was given an excruciating pelvic examination, a shot of Demerol (a narcotic analgesic), and a prostaglandin inhibitor to slow down her contractions. Then after mild bleeding for six more days, she hemorrhaged. She continued to bleed for three months. Tamara Keta Hodgson states that no one is sure why she had such an extreme response. She chose chemical abortion because it was presented to her as a 'relatively benign experience' and because she thought it would advance the causes of both women and science.

Do I think RU 486 should be licensed in the United States? I'm not sure. I had access to many resources not available to the general population of women who might take the drug. I am a registered nurse who works at one of the most sophisticated hospitals in the world. I was cared for by the research team investigating the drug. I had no children who needed to be cared for.

The same cannot be said for women of the Third World. It also cannot be said for women in the United States who do not have access to adequate health care (Hodgson in *Los Angeles Times*, 1990: E20).

RU 486/PG has tremendous problems for distribution in the third world and in areas of western countries where poor, Black, and other minority women may not have middle-class health care and facilities available. Yet much of the medical and feminist championing of RU 486 continues to promote it as a corrective for the 200,000 botched abortions which injure women worldwide, most of which are reported to happen in developing countries.

Some supporters of RU 486 have questioned its use in third world countries, but mostly in the context of cost. Commenting on the need for ß-hCG and ultrasound testing in the Grimes trials in Southern California, Allan Rosenfield states:

> This will be a question of particular importance, given the cost involved, for clinics serving the poor and for programs in developing countries . . . Similarly, I would like his [Grimes] comment on the routine use of ultrasonography before prescribing the drug. He mentions that vaginal ultrasonography to rule out fetal cardiac activity is now a standard procedure in his program . . . Again, of course, there are cost implications of this recommendation for general use (Rosenfield in Grimes *et al.*, 1990: 916).

Edouard Sakiz, chairman of Roussel Uclaf, in an interview in the French daily, *Le Monde*, has stated quite explicitly:

> Our idea was to market the product in those developed countries which have the same legislation on abortion as

France, and which are equally keen to use the product. Now you have to remember there aren't many countries that fit the bill, particularly as we insist on there being the same very tight distribution controls as we have here in France. Here, a doctor can write out a prescription for a narcotic drug, but he [*sic*] can't prescribe RU 486. That can only be done through an authorised clinic, and the name of the patient has to be registered. (Nau, 1990: 16).

What happened to all those women who could benefit from RU 486 in the developing countries? What happened to the privacy claims for RU 486? Furthermore, RU 486/PG is contraindicated for vast numbers of women, and its list of complications pose unacceptable hazards for all women.

Contraindications

When one examines the criteria used to admit women to the RU 486/PG trial protocols, one finds numerous conditions that exclude large numbers of women from chemical abortion treatment. First, the majority of studies recommend that chemical abortion is only suitable for women 18 years of age or older (e.g. Sitruk-Ware *et al.*, 1985: 245; Swahn and Bygdeman, 1989: 293; Grimes *et al.*, 1988: 1307). This age recommendation excludes teenagers between 13 and 17, a group that proponents of chemical abortion argue could benefit from its alleged gentler effects, as compared with the alleged harsher effects of conventional abortion. The upper age limit is poorly defined in the studies with recommendations for women up to 35 years of age (WHO Trial, 1989a: 719); women up to 40 years of age (Swahn and Bygdeman, 1989: 293); or women up to 42 years of age (Couzinet *et al.*, 1986: 1565). In 1991, the French Health Ministry restricted RU 486/PG abortion to women who are younger than 35 years of age. These age restrictions exclude a considerable number of women.

Second, the effectiveness of RU 486/PG abortion is

limited by the actual age of the woman's pregnancy. This too is poorly defined with some studies proposing a cut-off pregnancy age of 42 days (e.g. Gao *et al.*, 1988: 676; Maria *et al.*, 1988: 255), but with the larger number of studies advocating an outer limit of 49 days (e.g. Somell and Ölund, 1990: 13; Zheng, 1989: 19). Trials conducted in England included women who were pregnant for up to 56 days (Roger and Baird, 1987: 1415; Cameron and Baird, 1988: 272) or, as in the UK Multicentre Trial, 63 days (1990: 481).

There are a multitude of other contraindications, many relating to a woman's menstrual and reproductive history. Women with evidence of menstrual irregularities are excluded from some trials. 'Regularity' is defined as 28 days plus/minus three days (Couzinet *et al.*, 1986: 1565; Grimes *et al.*, 1988: 1307). Women with fibroids, abnormal menstrual bleeding, or endometriosis were not admitted to some studies (Li *et al.*, 1988: 733). 'Cervical incompetence' is another contraindication (Grimes *et al.*, 1988: 1307; and 1990: 911). Other studies exclude women with a previous abortion history, spontaneous or induced (Sitruk-Ware *et al.*, 1985: 243; Grimes *et al.*, 1990: 911). Past and/or present history of 'abnormal pregnancies' including multiple and ectopic pregnancies exempts a further number of women (Rodger and Baird, 1987: 1415; Sylvestre *et al.*, 1990: 645). Pelvic inflammatory disease (PID) excludes still more women (Couzinet *et al.*, 1986: 1565; Maria *et al.*, 1988: 250).

Some studies rule out women who have used IUDs or hormonal contraception three months prior to or during the last cycle in which conception occurred (Swahn and Bygdeman, 1989: 293; WHO Trial, 1989a: 719). The claim that RU 486/PG abortion is the safe treatment of choice for large numbers of women shrinks further in the light of the significant number of women worldwide who use either IUDs or the contraceptive pill. However, because only a few studies disallow contraceptive users from chemical abortion treatment, what awaits women who take the pill and then attempt chemical abortion? Will their risks be identified, or will there be further tragedies?

Still more women are excluded by their medical history. Any one of the following problems is sufficient grounds for non-treatment: allergies including asthma (Sylvestre *et al.*, 1990: 646); epilepsy (Cameron and Baird, 1986: 272); adrenal insufficiency (Sylvestre *et al.*, 1990: 645); kidney disease (Vervest and Haspels, 1985: 627); gastro-intestinal disorders (Maria *et al.*, 1988: 250); liver disorder (Couzinet *et al.*, 1986: 1565); pulmonary disorder (Somell and Ölund, 1990: 13); or simply a 'history of serious medical disorder' (Rodger and Baird, 1987: 1415).

The list of contraindications continues. Any woman who has taken steroid medication in the past 12 months (UK Multicentre Trial, 1990: 481), six months (Grimes *et al.*, 1988: 1306), three months (Maria *et al.*, 1988: 250) or 'recently' (Sitruk-Ware *et al.*, 1990: 223) is excluded. This exclusion is related to the antiglucocorticosteroid properties of RU 486/PG (see Chapter Three).

More critically, some *non-steroidal* medications may serve to reduce the effectiveness of the PG component of RU 486/PG abortion. Anti-inflammatory medication, as well as simple aspirin, are known prostaglandin inhibitors. Therefore, their simultaneous use with RU 486/PG almost guarantees that the abortion will be incomplete. This means that women have two poor alternatives (not choices!): narcotic analgesics or suffering pain that may be intolerable.

Finally, in light of the documented accidents and death from RU 486/PG abortions linked to cardiovascular complications, we were astonished to find that only a few studies excluded women on the basis of such cardiovascular criteria (e.g. Cameron and Baird, 1988: 272). Sylvestre *et al.*, (1990: 646) exclude women who have a history of hypertension and/or clotting disorders. Smoking was not included in the contraindications of studies from 1985 to 1990, but this may change following the Roussel Uclaf warnings from April 1990 and confirmed by the April 1991 French woman's death blamed on cardiovascular complications caused by 'heavy smoking'.

Increasingly, there are more and more contraindications added to the list. Obesity is now identified as an additional factor detracting from the RU 486/PG success rates (Vervest and Haspels, 1985: 627; Cameron and Baird, 1986: 273; WHO Trial, 1989a: 722; Grimes *et al.*, 1990: 913). More conditions will certainly be added in the future, restricting RU 486/PG to a further diminished population of women.

Complications

In a comprehensive review of medical journal articles, we examined and analyzed complications of chemical abortions. These articles covered a span of seven years (1984–90), and included the most well-known as well as some of the lesser known research. Because these studies have different criteria for measuring success, efficacy, and complications, and because they often use different protocols within the same study, it is difficult to ascertain patterns and an agreed-upon system of evaluation.

The difficulty starts with the *definition of age of pregnancy*. Most researchers would agree that RU 486, when used alone, or when used in combination with prostaglandins, works best when the pregnancy is less than 42–49 days. There is a disparity in how the 42–49 days figure is arrived at, since some researchers count from the first day of the last menstrual period (Swahn and Bygdeman, 1989); some are not specific, merely stating 42–49 days since the last menstrual period (Somell and Olund, 1990; and Grimes *et al.*, 1988); and some count from the expected onset of the last *missed* menstrual period, in which case there are only approximately 14–21 days when RU 486/PG is operational (see Couzinet *et al.*, 1986). Since timing is critical to an RU 486/PG abortion, the exact age of pregnancy is crucial.

There is, however, at least one study that maintains that

the age of pregnancy has no significant effect, provided that it is less than 43 days, on the outcome of treatment (Sitruk-Ware *et al.*, 1990). Additionally, most researchers now contend that ultrasound or measurement of ß-hCG levels are more reliable indicators of the age of pregnancy than a woman's testimony regarding her own menstrual cycle. If ultrasound becomes the preferred measure of assessing the age of pregnancy, this may result in more complications in third world countries where the equipment may not be available.

Incomplete abortions with or without a continuing pregnancy constitute the second complication. In studies where RU 486 is used without prostaglandin analogues, incomplete abortions/continuing pregnancies ranged from 44 per cent (Kovacs, 1984) to 10 per cent (Grimes *et al.*, 1988). Where a combination of RU 486/PG is used, in the more recent clinical studies, incomplete abortions/ continuing pregnancies ranged from 13.4 per cent (Gao *et al.*, 1988) to two per cent (Rodger and Baird, 1989). However, one woman in this last-mentioned study required emergency surgery. Incomplete abortions and ongoing pregnancies, of course, necessitate that the products of conception are removed by conventional abortion methods. Incomplete evacuation can be accompanied by severe bleeding due to tissue that remains in the cervical area and is usually remedied by dilation and curettage. One study indicated that a woman who had been classified as a success returned two months later because of residual decidual material (Sitruk-Ware *et al.*, 1990: 228). This adverse effect of RU 486/PG abortion may lead to other possible complications such as pelvic inflammatory disease (PID) from infection, to infertility, and possibly uterine cancer.

In one study, clinicians administering RU 486 without prostaglandin analogues 'adopted a conservative approach with weekly ß-HCG and ultrasound evaluation.' They reported that 29 out of 124 women did not terminate their pregnancies until 'between Day 15 and Day 45 after commencing therapy.' This is an extremely long and unacceptable period of time that women must wait to abort (Sitruk-Ware *et al.*, 1990: 227–28).

A 1990, as yet unpublished Roussel Uclaf study indicates that 4.7 per cent of 10,250 women had incomplete abortions, with or without continuing pregnancies, after RU 486/PG treatment. A percentage is abstract; the less abstract fact is that this 4.7 per cent constitutes 482 real women for whom chemical abortion not only failed, but who then had to submit to an additional abortion procedure (Aubeny, 1990:3). Translated into the raw truth of human data, the RU 486/PG failure rate is by no means minimal.

Bleeding is another area of complication. In several studies, some women were reported to receive blood transfusions. The largest number of transfusions reported in the literature took place in the UK Multicentre studies where five out of 579 women required both blood transfusions and curettage (UK Multicentre Trial, 1990: 482). Sometimes, heavy bleeding necessitates an emergency uterine evacuation; other times, when a uterine evacuation is performed because of an incomplete RU 486 abortion, the evacuation itself leads to heavy bleeding (Cameron *et al.*, 1986: 463).

More commonly, studies chronicle bleeding in terms of its duration and volume. Many articles report severe and prolonged blood loss. Duration of bleeding ranges from one to 44 days (Rodger and Baird, 1989). The 1990 UK Multicentre Trial mentions that the mean duration of bleeding experienced by women was almost two weeks.

Severe or excessive bleeding, as opposed to duration, is reported in conjunction with treatment regimens. In one study after administration of RU 486, nine per cent of women experienced heavy bleeding; and when the prostaglandins were subsequently administered as the second medication in the treatment, another nine per cent bled heavily. Two days after the completion of the combination treatment, 16 per cent reported heavy bleeding (UK Multicentre Trial, 1990: 483). In many other studies, prolonged heavy bleeding is regarded as the chief problem and most serious side-effect of chemical abortions (Couzinet *et al.*, 1986; Grimes *et al.*, 1988).

Some researchers have attempted to make distinctions between the severity of bleeding caused by RU 486 when used alone, and that due to RU 486 in combination with prostaglandins. Couzinet *et al.* report that the chief problem with RU 486 administration was the prolonged heavy bleeding in 18 per cent of the women. They suggest that the addition of 'a small dose of prostaglandin' might be effective in limiting excessive bleeding (Couzinet *et al.*, 1986: 1569). Bygdeman and Swahn contend in several studies that the combination treatment may decrease the severity of bleeding (e.g. Swahn and Bygdeman, 1989: 298). However, the WHO Multicenter study cites one center with an 'unacceptably high frequency of heavy bleeding' when combined treatment is used. Thus they conclude that 'It is therefore questionable whether the risk of heavy bleeding is diminished by using a combination of these two substances' (Swahn and Bygdeman, 1989: 298). Another study by Cameron *et al.* (1986) had arrived at a similar conclusion.

In the first Chinese Multicenter study, 23 per cent of 160 women were reported to have 'subjectively' experienced heavy bleeding (Gao *et al.*, 1988). In this study, oral contraceptives were used to stop the bleeding 'in some cases' (no exact number given). In other studies, women were prescribed oral contraceptives after completion of the abortion so that the bleeding may have been stopped artificially (Sitruk-Ware *et al.*, 1990). In studies where heavy bleeding is reported, the range of those experiencing heavy bleeding falls between 15–25 per cent. *Ob. Gyn. News* reports 'The average blood loss is about 70 cc, about equal to two average menstrual periods. In contrast, blood loss with suction curettage is limited to 10–20 cc in early abortions . . . '(*Ob. Gyn. News*, 1989: 1).

Some studies cite differences between severe and moderate bleeding. In the Chinese Multicenter Trial (Gao *et al.*, 1988), 23 per cent of the women experienced heavy bleeding and 67.8 per cent reported moderate bleeding. Other studies mention that bleeding was significant enough to cause loss of work. One study notes that although blood loss was not life-threatening, it could compromise the health of women in a population in which anemia is endemic, as in many developing countries (Rodger and Baird, 1989: 445). Many studies report a significant drop in hemoglobin levels. A critical drop in hemoglobin, which is a decrease in the oxygen-carrying capacity of the body's red blood cells, leads to low blood pressure and shock and often necessitates a blood transfusion. In one study, 15.3 per cent of women had almost a 10 per cent fall in their hemoglobin levels (Sitruk-Ware *et al.*, 1990). Sixteen out of 150 women were prescribed iron therapy to repair the hemoglobin deficit (Maria *et al.*, 1988).

Contradictorily, studies reporting bleeding as a significant side-effect of the treatment also state that it is not excessive (Grimes *et al.*, 1988). Other studies distinguish between moderate and mild bleeding (Hill *et al.*, 1990a). Rodger and Baird state quite baldly: 'As we gained experience, we became more confident in disregarding minimum continued vaginal bleeding' (Rodger and Baird, 1987: 1417).

The disregarding of these factors by researchers establishes the standards which determine the acceptability of different degrees of blood loss; severe versus moderate versus mild. Judgements about the seriousness of bleeding, like judgements about the severity of pain, are in the subjective/objective eye of the beholder. It becomes clear that complications, such as bleeding and pain, are often evaluated differently by researchers than by women themselves. 'Pain is a difficult parameter to compare, as the perception of pain by the individual and supervisory personnel depends on social and cultural factors, as well as availability of analgesics' (Swahn and Bygdeman, 1989: 298–99).

The message here is that women and medical personnel in different cultures and in different social contexts will react differently to pain. In assessing the degree of pain as a complication in these studies, we found that we had to address the perception of pain and who was perceiving it. In most studies, the dominant evaluator of pain is that of the medical 'culture' which often minimizes women's pain, reporting it as 'insignificant,' 'acceptable,' and/or 'tolerable.' Almost all studies, whatever the protocol, report that women experience pain, but most often classify it as mild to moderate. When PGs are added, severe pain is more frequently reported in combination with other gastro-intestinal side effects. However, this pain and gastro-intestinal effects are often attributed to the pregnancy itself. '. . . it is difficult to determine if these symptoms are related to the drug administration or to the pregnancy itself' (Ulmann *et al.*, 1987: 278).

More recent studies often compare the pain of combined RU 486/PG with pain experienced after the use of PGs alone (e.g. Silvestre *et al.*, 1990: 647). This is an outrageous comparison since many researchers have candidly stated that the use of PGs alone for abortion is intolerable because of the associated pain (see Chapter Four). A more honest assessment of pain would be to compare RU 486/PG termination to the pain of conventional abortion, not to a treatment that has been largely abandoned because of its extremely painful effects (Zheng, 1989: 19).

The unarticulated message about pain in many of these studies is that female pain is expected. Pain is reported by most women, but more and more pain is interpreted as less and less, because the threshold for female pain is constantly raised. For example, many of the women in these studies experienced pain for several days/weeks until the abortion was complete. Thus we are talking about prolonged, not transient pain, although this is rarely noted. Much of the medical journal commentary on pain dismisses it in one brief breeze of a sentence. Some articles provide details of the painful treatment effects but nonetheless still dismiss women's pain as minor or insignificant. Women who have had children – referred to as multiparous women – are reported to experience much less pain than nulliparous women, i.e. women who have not had children. The implication here is that, like the traditional perception of menstrual cramps, once a woman has a child the pain disappears; or the woman herself won't complain as much, having already gone through the pains of labor. Ultimately, to be a woman means to have some degree of pain and, for women then, pain is almost an ontological reality, writ large in gynecological and obstetrical situations. Both severe and moderate pain are thus perceived as normal and natural by the researchers and often by the women themselves. The medical studies accept without comment or criticism, the facticity of some kind of pain. Pain that would be unnatural/intolerable for men is natural/tolerable for women.

Another way of minimizing the degree of pain is to compare the pain from RU 486/PG treatment to that of menstrual cramps. The implication here is that menstrual cramps are 'minimal,' 'tolerable,' and 'acceptable' and because many women experience cramps, the pain of treatment is insignificant. However, many women's menstrual cramps are severe – not minimal – so the acceptance of this standard of comparison reiterates the cultural perception that women experience constant monthly pain anyway, so what is a degree more?

One way of noting the disparity between reported standards of 'minimal' pain and the degree of actual pain is the percentage of analgesics given to women in these studies. Most women are given some kind of painkiller, but a significant number are given opiate or narcotic analgesics, often by intramuscular injection (see Chapter Four for analgesics appropriate for use with RU 486/PG abortions). In the UK Multicentre Trial of 579 women, eight to 50 per cent required narcotic analgesia. An additional 30 per cent required non-narcotic analgesia (UK Multicentre Trial, 1990: 483). Another single-center British study reported that 23 per cent of 100 women were given opiate analgesia (Hill *et al.*, 1990a: 414). A Swedish study reported that 16 per cent of 160 women were given an injectable painkiller. This study was broken down into four sub-groups, and in two of the sub-groups, the percentages were as high as 25 and 30 per cent (Swahn and Bygdeman, 1989).

In the largest published multicenter study to date reporting on treatment with 2,040 women in France (75 women who did not return for follow-up were excluded from the study), only one per cent required opiate analgesia. The novel feature of this study, however, was that in one of the sub-groups of 378 women who were given 0.5 mg of the prostaglandin, sulprostone, 76 per cent were premedicated (the study does not specify what the premedication was). This adds a new twist on the recording of pain since premedication dulls women's perception and experience of pain to follow. Therefore, one would speculate that the amount of pain reported by these women would be lower. In spite of the premedication, however, 51.2 per cent of the 378 women who were premedicated still required further analgesia (Silvestre *et al.*, 1990: 648).

The assessment of gastrointestinal side-effects presents a special problem. Some studies treat vomiting, nausea, and diarrhea as a single side-effect. Some assess them separately. It is generally claimed that the addition of PGs to the treatment regimen leads to vomiting, nausea, and diarrhea, and therefore some studies give figures before and after PG administration. Where these three gastrointestinal complications are not separated, figures in the combination treatment studies are in the 20 per cent range (Gao *et al.*, 1988). Zheng reports vomiting and nausea together, citing a 48.3 per cent occurrence in 97 women (Zheng, 1989: 22). When reported separately, figures for vomiting range from 18 per cent out of 116 women (nine per cent after RU 486 administration and nine per cent after PG (Swahn and Bygdeman, 1989); to 15.3 per cent out of 2,040 women (Silvestre *et al*, 1990). Figures for nausea range from 57 per cent of 70 women (Somell and Ölund, 1990) [this is the mean figure of women experiencing nausea complications in both the failure and the success group, since the study differentiates]; to 25 per cent of 100 women (Hill *et al*, 1990a: 414). Figures for diarrhea range from 13 per cent out of 579 women (UK Multicentre Trial); to 8.2 per cent of 97 women (Zheng, 1989).

For regimens using RU 486 without PG analogues, gastrointestinal effects remain significant, despite the claims that it is the addition of PGs which promotes these complications. Zheng, who combined nausea and vomiting statistics cites 40 per cent out of 95 women who experience both (Zheng, 1989). Grimes reports vomiting as occurring in 14 per cent of those who aborted and in 60 per cent of those women who did not abort. Figures for nausea range from 27 per cent of 124 women (Sitruk-Ware *et al*, 1990); to 24 per cent of 100 women (Couzinet *et al*, 1986). Diarrhea is not a frequent complication after RU 486 administration unaccompanied by prostaglandin analogues.

If the reader is confused, it is because the studies are confusing. One impression, however, is prevalent. Gastrointestinal complications, and the range of such, are significant. The complications of vomiting and nausea seem unrelated to PGs, whereas diarrhea is mostly linked to PG administration in the combination treatment. Cameron *et al*, (1986), for example, report a low incidence of diarrhea with RU 486 alone (one per cent of 20 women).

Other immediate complications associated with chemical abortions are fainting (4.8 per cent in Sitruk-Ware *et al*, 1990); and fatigue (61.3 per cent in Sitruk-Ware *et al*, 1990).

Li *et al.* report a 23 per cent shift in mood change, manifesting itself as irritability and depression. They also report one case of marked thirst sensation. They thus conclude that the findings in their study demonstrate that RU 486 'affected the various functions of the hypothalamus' (Li *et al.*, 1988; see also Chapter Three).

Finally, Sitruk-Ware *et al.* cite the use of antibiotics both before and after vacuum aspiration with women who had incomplete abortions. They report that 25 per cent of the 28 women in their study who had incomplete abortions also developed a fever (Sitruk-Ware *et al.*, 1990). The question needs to be asked how many women who had incomplete abortions in other studies developed infections and fever and required antibiotics.

Promoters of RU 486/PG abortions emphasize their low percentage of complications. As we have demonstrated, this is not true. However, even where complications are of low incidence, in terms of percentages, it is important to ask how many women we are talking about. One percent of 579 women – the percent of women receiving blood transfusion in the UK Multicentre Trial – does in fact mean five women. Although too few women to acquire statistical significance, there is another standard we should employ here. Five women is five too many women. More critically, the number of women who might require transfusions in places where there is no medical backup to stop the bleeding and administer a transfusion could be significantly larger.

Ultimately, we must highlight the number of drugs that are now part of the chemical abortion treatment regimen because we view this as another complication. Nowhere has this melange of drugs been acknowledged. In light of the claims made that RU 486 is a simple, pill-popping method of abortion, we highlight the complexity, in cumulative fashion, of what has now become a drug cocktail.

In the beginning, there was:

1. RU 486
    Then, the researchers and clinicians added:
2. RU 486 + PG
    Then, the studies begin to cite:
3. RU 486 + PG + narcotic and other analgesics
    Then came the addition of:
4. RU 486 + PG + analgesics + pre-medication
    Finally, we read of:
5. RU 486 + PG + analgesics + pre-medication + antibiotics.

In some cases, oral contraceptives have also been used to stop bleeding, and anti-diarrhea and anti-nausea medications for the gastro-intestinal side-effects have been given to women.

The history of the development and application of chemical abortion has been an increasing regimen of drug cocktails. This is nothing new, of course, and has been part of the history of new reproductive medicine in general where all sorts of drug combinations, as well as ancillary medical procedures, are part of, for example, in vitro fertilization treatment (Klein/Rowland, 1988).

Researchers and clinicians minimize the drug cocktail effect, as they minimize other complications. As we evaluated the literature on complications, it became clear to us that the medical acceptance, without comment or criticism, of what have now become 'minimal,' 'tolerable,' and 'acceptable' side effects for women – deserves to be highlighted for what it is – unethical medical practice. In conclusion, this point can best be illustrated by quoting a typical example of 'acceptable' side-effects in one test group.

Six patients had an incomplete abortion and in one the pregnancy continued unaffected. Side effects included intense uterine pain after the prostaglandin administration (16%), vomiting associated with the antiprogestin intake (9%) and after the prostaglandin administration (9%). One woman needed emergency curettage due to heavy bleeding. Six percent of the treated patients had a decrease in hemoglobin exceeding 20 g/l during the first week but no patient needed blood transfusion. *No serious side effects were recorded* (Swahn and Bygdeman, 1989: 293, emphasis ours).

Chemical Abortion versus Conventional Abortion

Proponents of RU 486/PG abortions claim that chemical pregnancy terminations are safer than conventional abortions. However, there have been no systematic comparisons between RU 486/PG terminations, and conventional abortions performed by vacuum aspiration or surgical dilation, curettage, and evacuation. Various medical journal articles make mention of brief and generalized differences in the two methods, without noting that the category 'surgical abortion' is hardly monolithic or, for that matter, always surgical. Any comparison between RU 486/PG abortions and other conventional methods of abortion must take as its starting point a delineation of the various methods that are lumped into the imprecise category of surgical abortion.

Often, what are referred to as surgical methods are more appropriately termed suction methods. The medical articles focused on RU 486/PG abortions omit any discussion of the various methods of conventional abortion, an omission that is obfuscating and/or misleading. Routine first-trimester abortions fall into several categories: more surgical abortions performed by dilation and surgical curettage, and usually involving a general anaesthetic; less surgical vacuum aspiration abortions and other suction methods involving curettage, but usually employing a local anaesthetic.

Distinguishing between types of conventional abortions is crucial since promoters of RU 486/PG abortions are now routinely using the terminology of surgical as opposed to chemical abortions. One of the most frequently-cited differences between these two methods, so defined, is that RU 486/PG abortions avoid the traumas and dangers of surgery and anesthesia. With many conventional abortions, a general anaesthesic is not administered. Local anaesthesia is often given with suction abortion and/or vacuum aspiration so that the so-called risk of general anaesthesia, which many RU 486/PG promoters cite, is not at issue.

How comparisons are framed in the medical literature is a fascinating subject. When proponents of the RU 486/PG method compare it to the specious category, 'surgical abortion,' they raise doubts about the safety and invasiveness of the latter. In a brief comparison of RU 486/PG versus 'surgical' methods of abortion, two Swedish researchers state: '. . . avoiding the risk for cervical injury and other complications associated with surgical methods for termination of pregnancy is an advantage. Another important factor in favor of mifepristone is the low intrusion on personal integrity offered by this method' (Somell and Ölund, 1990: 15). Likewise, Couzinet *et al.* contend: '. . . RU 486 offers a reasonable alternative to surgical abortion, which carries the risks of anaesthesia, surgical complications, infertility, and psychological sequelae' (1986: 1569).

On the other hand, when surgical abortion is discussed in the context of criticizing the 1989 US Supreme Court's Webster v Reproductive Health Services decision, which granted states the right of regulation and restriction, surgical abortion is touted as '. . . one of the most scrutinized surgical procedures and has been demonstrated to be one of the safest' (Chavkin and Rosenfield, 1990: 451). We hear, in this context, about the almost-zero mortality rate associated with surgical abortion and about its significantly lower risk to women than childbirth. The ideology that abortion is dangerous and has risky complications is refuted in the context of assaults from the anti-abortionists, but asserted in the context of promoting RU 486/PG.

Women may justifiably ask why we hear about the supposed risks of conventional abortion only in the RU 486 literature. Right-to-Lifers are not so laid back. For example, Nuala Scarisbrick, administrator of Life, the British anti-abortion organization, said she was 'very amused that the researchers were coming clean about the dangers of abortion' in singing the praises of RU 486 over the regular surgical abortion procedure (*Sunday Times*, 30 October 1988). Such a misrepresentation of risks, when used by the promoters of RU 486/PG abortions in comparison to those of conventional terminations, can only aid and abet the anti-abortion movement.

The 'dangers of surgical abortion' strategy used by the pro-RU 486/PG lobby and literature deserves comment on other grounds as well. In the brief comparisons that have been made between chemical and conventional methods of abortion in the medical literature, proponents of RU 486/PG maintain that it avoids the risks of surgery and anaesthesia; is 95 per cent effective; requires little medical intervention; has few and minimal complications; and results in a small percentage of incomplete abortions (numbers vary in different various studies from five to 40 per cent depending on treatment regimens). They minimize the duration of bleeding (one to 44 days) which in a substantial percentage of women has been moderate (67%) to severe (23%); the occurrence of nausea, diarrhea, vomiting, dizziness, and fatigue frequently dismissed as pregnancy-related; the decrease in blood pressure; and the often strong uterine pain which regularly requires narcotic and injectable analgesics.

The overall impression conveyed in these brief comparisons is that the monolithic 'surgical' abortion is indeed dangerous and complicated. However, conventional abortions, as we have noted, do not largely involve surgical methods and general anaesthesia; are 99 per cent effective; require two medical visits as opposed to three or four for chemical abortions; have fewer contraindications and fewer and more minimal complications, result in fewer than one per cent incomplete abortions, and can be performed over a wider range of time. Even Edouard Sakiz, chairman of Roussel Uclaf, admits that:

> As abortifacient procedures go, RU 486 is not at all easy to use. In fact it is much more complex to use than the technique of vacuum extraction. True, no anaesthetic is required. But a woman who wants to end her pregnancy has to 'live' with her abortion for at least a week using this technique. It's an appalling psychological ordeal (Nau, 1990:16).

The length of time for a chemical abortion to 'take,' added to the time involved in multiple visits to the center of administration, is one great omission from the comparative assertions. Often a woman has to wait hours or days, or in some cases, weeks, for the embryo to be expelled. While this may not be 'an appalling psychological ordeal,' as Sakiz has termed it, at the very least it is an unpleasant and unwanted experience. In the meantime, bleeding has begun as well. Does the woman continue her work, or does she wait for the expulsion to happen in the privacy of her home or the 'privacy' of the street? Comparatively, conventional abortion has the advantage of being quick and time-limited, instead of multi-stepped and long drawn-out.

RU 486/PG works best within a 49-day time period after a woman's last period; conventional abortions can be performed safely and effectively within the entire first trimester of pregnancy. The RU 486/PG method is associated with greater blood loss than is suction curettage. Both, as delivered within the current medicalized setting, require doctor supervision. Physicians, however, are not necessary to perform conventional abortions, as we argue in the conclusion to this report. A trained lay practitioner is capable of performing skilled conventional terminations. While some methods of conventional abortion can lead to infection and uterine perforation, this depends on the method employed, the skill of the provider, and the context in which it is performed.

The abysmal safety statistics from conventional abortions in third world countries are often cited in defense of chemical abortion. But the RU 486/PG method is as unacceptable in these countries for the same reasons as poorly performed conventional abortions – lack of trained personnel and supervision. Moreover, in many third world countries, abortion is illegal. Many promoters of RU 486/PG are concerned about the effects of infection from conventional abortions done on women in developing countries, but seem unfazed by the possibilities of incomplete abortions, bleeding, and infection of women in these very same countries who won't have access to the medical supervision required by the RU 486/PG combination treatment.

The benefits and liabilities of these chemical and conventional methods – for doctors, hospitals, and the state – are another omission in the comparative literature. The cost of RU 486/PG abortion, for example, is not cheaper for *women*, but is much cheaper for the hospitals and clinics. Under the state security system in France, women are reimbursed the same amount (80%) whether it is a conventional or chemical abortion. For abortions that are performed in hospitals and that involve surgery or aspiration equipment and an operating room – as opposed to giving a woman pills and injectables/suppositories – there is a great difference in cost. The UK Women's Health and Reproductive Rights Information Centre *Newsletter* reports that the NHS (National Health Service) in Britain will save £15–20 million per year when England begins to use RU 486/PG and asks: 'In particular, if it is cheaper to administer RU 486 in the early states of pregnancy than perform a surgical abortion, are women to be denied surgical abortion if they choose this method on the NHS?' (*Newsletter*, 1990: 15–16)

Equally important for medical administrators and personnel is the liberating of these facilities for other medical procedures. 'As well as avoiding the risks of surgery and anaesthesia, medical treatment can be given on an outpatient basis and may thus free ward and theatre facilities, with obvious resource implications' (Urquhart and Templeton, 1988: 106).

Another consideration is the attitude of doctors toward conventional abortions. Many doctors resent or resist performing abortions. As has been documented in some studies, there is also a level of provider 'burn-out' in the delivery of conventional abortion services. Given this situation, it is not surprising that doctors may prefer chemical abortions over conventional methods because RU 486/PG actually humanizes the abortion experience more for the *doctor* than for the woman.

Providers' attitudes toward methods of abortion may have significant influence on the method selected by women. Many of the studies supporting the safety and effectiveness of RU 486/PG cite high percentages of women's satisfaction with this abortion technique. In the few follow-up questionnaires and/or interviews conducted after RU 486/PG treatment, women report 60–90 per cent preference for chemical over the indiscriminately termed 'surgical' method. Reasons such as 'awareness of what was happening to them,' 'more natural,' 'avoidance of general anaesthesia,' 'more discreet,' and 'less traumatizing' have all been mentioned. Perhaps because of women's experience of a prior anaesthetized surgical pregnancy termination, the climate of provider punitiveness toward women undergoing abortion, including doctors' ambivalence/ hostility to conventional methods, and the ways in which a larger social climate induces guilt in women who consider undergoing abortions, this preference is understandable. This is not to claim that conventional abortion is a positive and uplifting experience for women, nor that being in the stirrups promotes any version of female control. It is to say that RU 486/PG does not change this order of things.

An unfortunate effect of the brief comparisons offered in the medical journals between chemical and conventional abortions is that RU 486 can be pitted against suction and vacuum aspiration. Although many groups promoting RU 486/PG abortion regard it as a medical alternative for early pregnancy interruption, or as expanding the choices for women seeking abortion, some groups see it as the treatment of primary choice, or as a replacement for conventional abortion. 'Surgical abortion must now be regarded as obsolete in the light of the latest trials of the French "abortion pill"' (David Healey, quoted in *The Age*, McIntosh, 1990: 5).

Making conventional abortion methods obsolete has been one of the unexamined consequences of promoting and privileging RU 486/PG abortion. Currently, in France, one-third of all abortions involve use of the abortion pill. If long-term debilitating consequences eventually result from this drug in later years, as happened with DES for example, women may have reached the point where conventional methods of abortion will no longer be widely or even marginally available. Since RU 486/PG abortions must be done within a 42–49 day time period after the last menstrual period, that time may become the accepted cut-off point after which abortion could be made illegal.

Moreover, if abortions of any type continue to be restricted to medical control, there may also be a dearth of doctors trained to perform them. Citing one possible effect of the Webster decision on obstetrics and gynecology education, Chavkin and Rosenfield predict:

> If performance of abortion is not regularly included in obstetrics and gynecology training programs, it is likely that as experience decreases, complications will again rise ... Instead of training obstetrics and gynecology residents to be competent at this surgical procedure, we may soon have to teach them once again to diagnose and treat sepsis and other complications of an unsafe abortion (Chavkin and Rosenfield, 1990: 451).

The assault on conventional abortion by the right-wing and religious conservatives in the United States and other countries has, of course, increased the fervor for an abortion method that is self-administered, safe, effective, and free from harassment. Unfortunately, RU 486/PG does not fulfill these criteria. What the present situation seems to have generated is a general system of misconceptions. It is a misconception that the woman has control of this method, and not the doctor. It is a another misconception that because RU 486 is a pill, the method is quick and easy. It is a further misconception that medical instruments are not used. And the greatest misconception is that the new abortion pill will create an abortion alternative for women that is free from the present threat of the right-wing. In reality, it may, in fact, have just the opposite effect of consolidating abortion procedures at even more restricted and controlled medical centers, and of ultimately diminishing the availability of safe, conventional abortion for women.

CHAPTER THREE

What is RU 486 and How Does It Work?

Press reports describe RU 486 as an 'abortion pill' whose action is that of an 'anti-hormone' blocking the production of progesterone in the woman's uterus at the receptor level. Because progesterone prepares the lining of the uterus (the endometrium) to support a pregnancy, researchers state that inhibiting its action will terminate a pregnancy, or prevent implantation of a fertilized egg. While this official but simplified statement is not entirely wrong, it misleads the layperson, including any woman considering chemical abortion as the means to end her pregnancy, to believe that the action of RU 486 in a woman's body is *confined* to the womb. These truncated descriptions convince the general public that those promoting RU 486 as a 'safe' abortifacient fully understand how this chemical substance works. The reality is that the action of RU 486 alone, and especially its interaction with prostaglandin, is complex and far from totally understood.

In order to fully understand the important implications of chemical abortion, we begin with some information about the hormonal events that take place in a woman's body before and after she ovulates, and if fertilization occurs. We describe the (supposed) action of RU 486 on pregnancy termination. Because of potential problems for women's health, we also explain o*ther*sites of RU 486 action in the human body and its effects on women's fertility, eggs and embryos, an area in which little research has been done. Additionally, we refer to other applications of the drug.

Hormonal Interactions

The most important centre in the human body for the production of hormones is an endocrine gland, the pituitary, located at the base of the brain. It is often referred to as the 'master gland' because together with the hypothalamus – a regulatory site for such basic functions as hunger, thirst, sleep, temperature control and the reproductive system – its anterior lobe produces many hormones that control other glands in the body. RU 486 interacts with both the hypothalamus and the pituitary and, as researchers admit, the relationship between the pituitary and the hypothalamus is 'poorly understood'. RU 486 interference with the hypothalamic-pituitary axis may thus have unexpected and possibly unnoted effects on the body's metabolism.

In the female body, the anterior pituitary produces gonadotropins called FSH (follicle stimulating hormone) and LH (luteinizing hormone). Each month FSH activates the ripening of one of the thousands of immature egg cells in the ovaries and LH prompts the respective ovarian follicle to release the ripe egg. Stimulated by this action, one of the follicular cell layers secretes estrogen and just before the egg is released from the ovary, the follicle also begins secreting *progesterone*. After ovulation, the empty follicle, called the corpus luteum, continues to secrete progesterone which, together with the continuing secretion of estrogen, readies the womb for an eventual pregnancy. Estrogen prepares the wall of the uterus for implantation and nutrition of the early embryo and progesterone causes glands in the uterine lining, the endometrium, to secrete embryo nourishing substances. If fertilization does indeed take place, that is, if the egg fuses with sperm, part of the early embryo called the trophoblast (which evolves into the placenta), will begin to release hCG. This in turn prompts the corpus luteum to continue the progesterone and estrogen production needed to establish and maintain a pregnancy.

Because RU 486 is described as an anti-progesterone, a closer look at progesterone is warranted. Progesterone is a steroid hormone secreted by the corpeus luteum, the adrenal glands and, in the case of an established pregnancy, the placenta. It acts on the lining of the uterus, the myometrium (smooth muscle of the uterus), the cervix, as well as the fallopian tubes, the vagina, the ovaries, the breasts and importantly, the hypothalamus. According to Etienne Baulieu, the function of progesterone in these latter organs 'is not well understood' (1989b: 1351). An editorial in the *New England Journal of Medicine*, discussing 'Progesterone Antagonism' related to RU 486 puts it even more strongly: 'Progesterone's influence on the central nervous system is poorly understood, but the hormone *appears to have* diverse effects on the hypothalamic-pituitary axis, respiratory centre, and perhaps cortical function' (Crowley, 1986: 1607; our emphasis). Progesterone has a thermogenic effect leading to an increase in body temperature. All of these functions, Crowley notes, are not well researched.

Progesterone is also involved in follicle development (perhaps directly affecting the follicle), and in the process of ovulation. However, in Baulieu's words: 'Folliculogenesis depends in part on intraovarian progesterone…The control of ovulation is poorly understood in the human' (1989b: 1351).

In 'non-pregnant women' (or 'normal' women as Baulieu calls them to distinguish them from 'pregnant' women; 1988a: 5), progesterone is the main product of the corpus luteum. It is, Crowley states '. . .itself a curious endocrine

organ, which is programmed for demise within a fortn
unless it is 'rescued' from this fate by a fertilized ovum
(1986: 1607).[1] In the case of a pregnancy, human chorionic
gonadotropin (hCG) as previously directed by the anterior
pituitary through secretion of luteinizing hormone (LH),
continues to stimulate the corpus luteum to secrete
progesterone. However, '. . . the mechanism of its
[progesterone] secretion during pregnancy is incompletely
understood' (*idem.*). Together with estrogen it '. . . appears
to be all that the gravid [pregnant] uterus requires for the
fertilized ovum to complete its development during the
initial six to eight weeks' (*idem.*). After that time the placenta
and the embryo/fetus produce their own sex steroids.

It is a misconception, however, to perceive the antiprogestin RU 486 as a 'new' concept in fertility control.
Since the first decade of this century, researchers have
been interested in the role of the corpus luteum with
regard to the viability of a woman's pregnancy. While it was
clearly established that the corpus luteum played no role
after the seventh week of gestation, its role as a source of
progesterone to nourish the embryo during the first seven
weeks of pregnancy was less clear cut.

It is a further misconception to believe that this research
took place in order to expand or improve women's 'choices'
to control their reproduction. Quite unmistakenly, the
concept evolved as a means of population control. More
than 20 years ago, the Center of Population Research of the
U.S. National Institutes of Health became interested in the
corpus luteum and called for research to determine whether
to find 'means to inhibit corpus luteum function is a
desirable goal'. The specific intention of such research was
to restrict population growth in countries that were judged
to be 'under-developed.' If successful, the method(s) could
be extended to groups in the United States, Black, Hispanic
and Native American Women (Department of Health,
Education and Welfare, NIH, USA, 1969).

By 1972, Arpad Csapo *et al*,[2] in St. Louis, Missouri, had responded to this call and identified the corpus luteum as being *indispensible* to the viability of a pregnancy during its initial seven weeks. To establish this finding, his experimentation was performed not *in vitro*, not in animals, but in 12 pregnant women. Three of these women were to have their ovaries removed because of ovarian cysts, and the other nine women wanted to undergo legal abortion and tubal ligation. With abdominal surgery a luteectomy (excision of the corpus luteum) was performed through an incision in the ovarian capsule over the corpus luteum. It was removed in its entirety. The women were then assigned to two groups according to the effect of the luteectomy on their pregnancy. Group 1 included the seven women who aborted, usually four to five days after the surgery, although the abortion '. . .was not invariably complete. In one case the detached placenta and in another, a placental residue had to be removed by curettage.' The mean pregnancy age in Group 1 women was 49 days, whereas in the five women in Group 2 who did not abort, it was 61 days. Csapo *et al* concluded, despite their own admission that the estimates of gestational age might be in error 'by as much as four weeks' that the

. . . indispensibility of the early human corpus luteum in pregnancy is not challenged by reliable clinical evidence. Additional efforts to examine the regulatory role of this gland and of its product, progesterone, appear fully justified. Successful interference with critical progesterone levels in the pregnant uterus either through reduced synthesis or transport, decreased availability of receptor sites, or increased *in situ* catabolism, are promising prospective measures of fertility control (1972: 1067).

We contend that it was these studies of Csapo *et al* – performed with total disrespect of women's integrity and well being – that provided the impetus for research that is today claimed to be new and groundbreaking. The unethical

procedures women were subjected to in Csapo *et al.*
experiments are astounding. In the mentioned study, nine
women intended to undergo an abortion. Even if none of
the three women with ovarian cysts are included in Group 1,
this means that the expectations of at least two of the nine
women were not met by the experimentation. Since the
article does not provide details about which group of
women included those with ovarian cysts, the number of
women whom the experimentation failed may have been
five of the nine, and since two of the seven induced
abortions were incomplete, necessitating curettage, it may
have been as many as seven of the nine women. Whatever
the actual number of women, this study formed the basis
for a further investigation (Csapo *et al.*, 1973). This next
experiment – equally abusive of women – again confirmed
the crucial importance of the corpus luteum for the first
seven weeks of pregnancy. Subsequent theorists have been
reluctant to acknowledge that concepts developed for
purpose of fertility regulation are based on the notions and
experiments of Csapo *et al.* This may be the reason why
Etienne Baulieu is credited with being the 'father' of the
abortion pill. Nonetheless, it may be strongly argued that
without this fundamental information, RU 486 and similar
agents which interfere with women's fertility could not
have reached their current stage of development.

How RU 486 Works

Both progesterone *and* estrogen are responsible
for establishing and maintaining an early pregnancy up to
eight weeks, but it is progesterone only which is 'targeted'
by RU 486. More precisely, according to Baulieu,
progesterone 'acts on the target cells by way of a
progesterone *receptor*, a hormone binding protein' (1989b:
1351). It is the action of these uterine receptors that the
steroid RU 486 blocks, thereby inhibiting the secretion of
progesterone. With regard to pregnancy interruption,

Baulieu believes that RU 486 takes the place of progesterone after which this hormone can no longer be secreted and the uterine lining begins to break down.[3] After the fertilized egg has become fully implanted (usually 10 to 14 days after fertilization, which means approximately 26–32 days since the woman's last period), it is no longer nourished by progesterone. As a consequence, hCG levels decrease. This leads to the dissolution of the corpus luteum (luteolysis). Progesterone no longer firms the cervix and the myometrium, making it potentially easier for an embryo to be expelled. In addition, as Baulieu puts it, 'probably' natural prostaglandins are released to start uterine contractions.

In 1987, researchers from Schering Research Laboratories, Berlin questioned this last claim of natural prostaglandin production. Working with two antiprogestins almost identical to RU 486 – ZK 98.734 and ZK 98.299 – they posit the opposite. Based on their research with guinea pigs, they found that anti-progestins *inhibit* secretion of natural prostaglandins (Elger *et al*, 1987: 91). This may explain why RU 486 alone has a 20–40 per cent failure rate. It would also explain why bleeding without expulsion has been observed in some cases up to 45 days after commencing treatment (Sitruk-Ware, 1990: 228). The fact that bleeding is not proof of a complete abortion is a serious shortcoming of chemical abortion. In France, this has led to mandatory check-ups, preferably with ultrasound, for every woman 10–14 days after RU 486/PG administration. Ultrasound detects fetal tissue remaining in the womb, which could indicate infection and/or a continuing pregnancy. In such cases the termination needs to be repeated by conventional vacuum aspiration or suction curettage.

Schering's theory is not the only explanation for failed chemical abortions. Régine Sitruk-Ware *et al* at the Hôpital Necker in Paris concluded that RU 486 only affected the *superficial* layer of the uterine lining (the decidua compacta) while the deeper layers (decidua spongiosa) and the chorionic villi remained intact after administration of the drug and thus continued to nourish the embryo. Sitru.. Ware suggested that this might explain why RU 486 is most effective in very early stages of a pregnancy, that is before day 29, or when the size of the conceptus (embryo) measured by its sac diameter is less than 10 mm. Such an early cut-off date severely limits the number of women who might use RU 486 with some assurance of success: it is highly unlikely that many women realize before day 29 following their last period that they might be pregnant.

Others maintain that gestational sac size and time since a woman's last period are less important than the drug regimen used and initial ß-hCG values in predicting chemical abortion outcomes (Grimes *et al.*, 1990). U.S. researcher David Grimes reached this conclusion after administering no less than 13 different treatment regimens to 271 women between July 1984 and January 1989. The multiplicity of drug protocols reflects how women are experimented upon in a trial-and-error fashion.

- Grimes *et al.* concluded that 600 mg per treatment – a very high dose –works best. This dosage coincides with that now commonly used in France. However, a WHO Multicenter Trial involving eight centers used multiple but significantly lower doses: 25 mg for three or four days (1989a). Paul van Look from the WHO Taskforce on Post-Ovulatory Methods for Fertility Regulation pointed out that '. . .these findings suggest that it may be possible to obtain the same rate of complete abortion with much lower doses of mifepristone than the 600 mg dose currently recommended by the manufacturer' (van Look, 1990: 3). Some other researchers state that success is independent of dosage, e.g. the study of Beatrice Couzinet *et al.* which used 400, 600 and 800 mg regimens (1986); and the study of Régine Sitruk-Ware *et al.* which used four different drug regimens (1990).

We therefore find it highly questionable that thousands of French women are now given a single drug dose of 600 mg whose short and long-term effects are far from being fully identified. It is, of course, simpler and quicker to administer a single dose. More important, administration of low doses spread over seven days would further shatter the myth that RU 486/PG abortion is an 'easy' and convenient way of terminating a pregnancy.

Both the WHO Multicenter Trial (1989) and the 1990 Grimes *et al.* summary mention yet another hypothesis for unsuccessful RU 486 abortion. According to Grimes: 'body mass appears to influence the likelihood of abortion with mifepristone' (1990: 910). In 'obese' women, Grimes *et al.* contend that RU 486 may be diluted because of their larger circulating blood volume. Alternatively, body fat may extract a high amount of the drug (i.e. make it unavailable for action in the uterine lining). However, the question is, what weight qualifies as obese? Grimes provides no figures, but the WHO paper lists women whose mean weight was 65.7 kg/145 pounds (no height correlation given) as those who have an increased likelihood of experiencing treatment failure (1989: 722). A weight of 65.7 kg is not unreasonable for medium-to-tall women. And if RU 486 administration is limited to thin or undernourished women, this further limits its general usefulness as an abortifacient. Grimes mentions that little is known about the influence of estrogen – produced by fatty tissue – on the action of RU 486. This raises another unanswered question: unaffected estrogen in the endometrium might convert RU 486 into a progesterone agonist, thereby inhibiting RU 486 activity.

Another unresolved question about RU 486 is its half-life.[4] (The term 'half-life' indicates the time taken for the activity of a substance to reduce to half its initial value.) Baulieu contends that the half-life of RU 486 in plasma is 12–24 hours after an intake of less than 200 mg. (Currently 600 mg are administered). He notes that, 'With a larger dose, the complex metabolic behaviour *is not fully understood,* but a single oral administration can create high plasma concentration *for several days*' (1989b: 1353; our emphasis).[5] Li *et al.* found the half-life of RU 486 to be 54 hours (1988)

and Sitruk-Ware *et al.* found that, 'Circulating levels wei
still detectable fourteen days after the last drug intake'
(1990: 232).

It is also known that: RU 486 is resorbed by fat and the
liver (Somell and Ölund, 1990), thus reducing its
bioavailability; it (and its metabolites) has been found in
pre-ovulatory follicles; as an antiglucocorticoid blocker it
affects the adrenal gland; as a progesterone blocker its
action is *not* restricted to the uterine lining; and it also acts
on the central nervous system (e.g. the hypothalamic-
pituitary-adrenal system and the respiratory center).[6] In
other words, the whereabouts of RU 486 and its metabolites
outside the blood stream are insufficiently known and data
about its half-life are contradictory.[7]

RU 486 chemistry further demonstrates that the drug
has *progesterone-like* properties. The chemical structure of
RU 486 reveals that it is a synthetic steroid derived from the
progesterone analogue norethindrone (norethisterone)
which is a synthetic analogue of progesterone. RU 486 is
called an 'anti- hormone' and its action to block the
progesterone receptor is explained as working as an
antagonist to progesterone. (It is also related to antiestrogens
such as tamoxifen which is a derivative of the synthetic
analogue of estradiol, diethylstilbestrol, DES). However,
Gravanis *et al.* (1985) administered RU 486 to postmenopausal women who had been given estradiol, and
concluded that it had some *pro*-gestational activity. This
means that RU 486 may also act as a progesterone *agonist*
(i.e. *similar* to progesterone). This finding was deemed
sufficiently significant to further investigate RU 486 as an
ovulation inhibitor and LH suppressor (i.e. as a
contraceptive) and for potential use as an anti-cancer drug
for people with estrogen-sensitive tumors who have become
resistant to tamoxifen. The unexplained mechanism of
this RU 486 effect questions its adverse effects stemming
from its potential progesterone-*like* qualities.

It has been specifically suggested that RU 486 does *not*

terminate ectopic pregnancies (e.g. by Etienne Baulieu on Radio New Zealand, Nov. 1990 and Levin *et al.*, 1990). The question must be asked could it perhaps *cause* them because of its progesterone-like properties? Progestagen-only contraceptive pills ('mini-pills') are known to cause an increased proportion of ectopic pregnancies (Kleinman, 1990: 60 and 64), due to their effect on the endometrium and ovarian function. Alternatively, RU 486 damage to fertilized eggs not yet implanted might cause ectopic pregnancies. Further, complete suppression of ovarian function and the appearance of ovarian cysts have been reported after progestagen-only pill use.[8] Promoters of chemical abortion assure us that its single administration cannot lead to the same problems that women have experienced with long-term contraceptives. However, this assumption is far from uncontested: reproductive functions may be irreversibly damaged, or irretrievably altered, by one single hormonal upheaval.

Cardiovascular risk is a further concern linked to the demonstrated progesterone-like nature of RU 486. The French Drug Evaluation Committee demanded that Roussel Uclaf issue stricter guidelines for RU 486/PG administration due to recently documented cardiovascular accidents. Numerous studies have demonstrated that the progestin component in oral contraceptives deregulates lipid metabolism (Kafrissen, 1990). This in turn increases atherosclerotic risk and cardiovascular disease (strokes, myocardial infarctions).[9] Further research into the effects of progesterone receptor blockade by RU 486 revealed degenerative vascular changes (e.g. a significant increase in small blood vessel width) which may explain the cases of heavy vaginal bleeding after RU 486 administration (Li *et al.*, 1988: 738). The promoters of RU 486 abortion do not acknowledge these potential dangers to women's health and lives, nor the even more widely recognized relationship between prostaglandins and cardiovascular risk (see Chapter Four).

Despite these numerous unanswered questions, thousands of women have already been given a drug, whose molecular mechanism and biochemical properties are not extensively researched, let alone understood. Once more, as with the contraceptive pill, DES, fertility drugs and hormone replacement therapy, healthy women are used as living test-sites for an 'exciting new drug' (Klein/ Rowland, 1988). In fact, as William Crowley put it in his editorial: 'Progesterone antagonists [such as RU 486] are likely to prove crucial to understanding the physiology of progesterone and unraveling its role in various pathophysiologic and neoplastic states' (1986: 1608). The question we must ask is: what is the price *women* have to pay for providing their bodies to 'unravel' the mysteries of progesterone?

Other Sites of Actions and Applications of RU 486

In addition to its antiprogesterone activities, RU 486 is also an antiglucocorticoid. Even Baulieu acknowledges that, 'RU 486 has *strong* antiprogesterone and *antiglucocorticoid* activities. . . [It is also] a *weak* antiandrogen' (1989b: 1352, our emphasis). A brief look at some further hormonal interactions will point out some consequences of these other sites of RU 486 action.

The anterior pituitary produces ACTH (adrenal-cortex-stimulating hormone) which, as its name suggests, stimulates the adrenal glands to produce *corticosteroids*.[10] Adrenal glands are endocrine glands located just above the kidneys and whose inner portion, the medulla, produces 'stress hormones' such as (nor)epinephrine. These steroid hormones regulate carbohydrate and protein metabolism and maintain the function of heart, lungs, muscles and kidneys. Steroid hormone production, including glucocorticoids, increases during stress, anxiety and injury. Cortisone, produced in the adrenal cortex and cortisol, into which cortisone can be converted to regulate blood pressure and to counter inflammation, are well known glucocorticoids. They are essential hormones which promote the conversion of proteins to glucose (blood sugar) and glycogen (the major carbohydrate, stored chiefly in the liver and in muscles). Glycogen converted to glucose is the main source of energy for human beings. Abnormal levels in the urine indicate diabetes or kidney disease. RU 486 has also been described as a weak antiandrogen blocker,[11] androgen being produced in the adrenal glands.

This triple action of RU 486 against progesterone, glucocorticoids and androgens in the adrenal glands, together with its effect on the uterine lining, is cause for concern. WHO representative, van Look, suggests that perhaps it could be the antiglucocorticoid activity of RU 486 which is the reason why the chemical given *alone* is not sufficient to induce abortion (1990: 3). Since the first clinical trial in Geneva (1982) the antiglucocorticosteroid activity of RU 486 has been confirmed in subsequent studies (e.g. Kovacs *et al.*, 1984; Gaillard *et al.*, 1984; Couzinet and Schaison, 1988). It appears that when RU 486 blocks the glucocorticoid receptor, the anterior pituitary produces ACTH via negative feedback which in turn stimulates the adrenal gland to produce cortisol. This leads to elevated levels of both ACTH and cortisol. But as the negative feedback in the hypothalamus-pituitary system is now blocked, further demand for cortisol cannot be fulfilled. As Healy and Hodgen hypothesize from their monkey studies, 'An RU 486-produced blockage of the cortisol receptor may prevent the usual glucocorticoid stress response...' (i.e. the production of cortisol) (1985: 137). In another experiment, eight of the 11 male subjects developed a severe, generalized body rash. The rash disappeared five to six days after RU 486 was discontinued. One man developed symptoms and signs consistent with the diagnosis of adrenal insufficiency. The symptoms disappeared after RU 486 was discontinued and dexamethasone was administered for two days (Laue *et al.*,

1990: 1477). Another research team, Nieman *et al.* (1985, expressed concern about glucocorticoid insufficiency, suggesting that due to measurement difficulties, RU 486 should be given 'in concert with careful evaluation for signs and symptoms of adrenal insufficiency' (p. 539). Fatigue, abdominal pain, nausea, dizzy spells or fainting, together with increased susceptibility to infection or physical stress, have been observed following prolonged steroid therapy.

Alarmingly, these are some of the symptoms mentioned by women after they have taken RU 486. Régine Sitruk-Ware *et al.*, in their small study of ten women given RU 486, questioned whether 'the asthenia [loss of energy] and weakness noted in all subjects represent subjective evidence of glucocorticoid deficiency' (1985: 247). Similarly, Healy and Hodgen ask if 'such an antiglucocorticoid effect may complicate anaesthesia and recovery' in the woman who 'needs curettage after an RU 486-induced abortion' (1985: 137). In other words, the health of the five to six per cent of women for whom RU 486/PG abortion fails may be further jeopardized during their second (conventional) abortion.

Baulieu maintains that no adverse effects result from blocking cortisol action at the hypothalamus-pituitary level. He further remarks that should any sign of cortisol insufficiency 'unfortunately' appear, it could easily be reversed by glucocorticosteroid administration (1985: 19). We contend this is another familiar example of bad medical practice where one drug's adverse effects are countered with the prescription of yet another. Baulieu suggests that 'the use of RU 486 in a provocative test for the exploration of the brain-pituitary-adrenal system may be of great interest to analyze some aspects of the neuroendocrine functioning...' (*idem.*). Provocative and of great interest for whom we might ask? Who gains laurels[12] and who pays the price?

The antiglucocorticosteroid property of RU 486 has led to the claim that it might be used in the treatment of Cushing's syndrome which is an overproduction of glucocorticoid hormones. The symptoms of Cushing's syndrome include muscular weakness, excessive hair growth, weight gain, high blood pressure, increased susceptibility to infections and, in later stages, diabetes. It can be caused by a tumor of the pituitary gland which produces too much ACTH, or after taking large doses of steroid drugs over a prolonged period. Isolated studies of RU 486 therapy give contradictory data: Nieman *et al.* (1985: 539) claim success in *one* male patient with severe Cushing's syndrome, despite his final fate of bilateral adrenalectomy. Bertagna *et al.* (1986) are more sceptical. Two of their seven patients developed headaches and nausea whilst another became lethargic. Administration of a glucocorticosteroid (dexamethasone) stopped these adverse effects within minutes (but dexamethasone has its own ill effects). The researchers concluded that the symptoms may have been due to glucocorticoid deprivation, but point out that it is extremely difficult 'to evaluate such a situation bio-chemically since cortisol measurements are of no value in a situation in which cortisol action is antagonized' (p. 642). We question whether the lack of evidence incriminating the antiglucocorticosteroid properties of RU 486 is due to the fact that there is no adequate technical means of measurement.

It is bemoaned that RU 486 is not freely available for research on and treatment of other conditions, e.g. glaucoma,[13] meningioma (brain tumor) and breast cancer. Each of these studies are in their initial stages and full of contradictions. In the case of meningioma, researchers have yet to agree which tumors are hormone dependent. One study reported further tumor growth during RU 486 administration (Blankenstein *et al.*, 1989).

In the case of breast cancer, Bardon *et al.* (1985) investigated the potential use of RU 486 to slow the growth of breast cancer progesterone-dependent cultured cell lines. Rather than preventing progesterone receptor activation, they found that RU 486 may work as a cytotoxic agent (a cell poison; see also Parinaud *et al.*, 1990; 1537 for a similar result in human cell culture). This raises a crucial question for the use of RU 486 as an abortifacient. If it is a cytotoxic drug, does RU 486 terminate pregnancies by non-specific cell poisoning? Such an explanation would be far removed from the current understanding of anti-progesterone activity. Another experiment found that the tumor-inhibiting potential of ZK 112.993 (a Schering drug) was greater than that of RU 486 (Schneider *et al.*, 1990: 683).

To end this section on other sites and applications of RU 486, it has also been administered to women on IVF programs whose pregnancies do not continue (Asch *et al.*, 1990: 481). This is the case for 20–40 per cent of women who had a successful embryo transfer. After fertility hormone cocktails, hormone monitoring and invasive egg harvesting procedures, they might now be administered yet another hazardous chemical: RU 486.

The Effect of RU 486 on Women's Menstrual Cycles, Fertility, Eggs and Embryos

Etienne Baulieu consistently extends the application of RU 486 beyond the drug's use as an abortifacient to other realms of female reproduction. As he puts it: 'RU 486 is a new medical tool for fertility control' (1988b: 127). Contraception is a case in point. Given at mid-cycle, RU 486 appears to delay ovulation. However, this feature would require continuous administration of the drug which, 'may be prohibited by the effects of chronically unopposed oestrogen on the endometrium' (Permezel, 1990: 78). In plain English, this means cancer of the endometrium may result, as it has with unopposed estrogen given to menopausal women.

Research to date, aimed at identifying possible uses of RU 486 as a means of fertility control before or after ovulation, reveals a host of contradictory data. The complexity of a woman's menstrual cycle and the many finely tuned interactions between ovaries, pituitary and hypothalamus are not fully understood. Nonetheless, researchers hope to tame the female reproductive cycle with the (anti)progesterone concept. Thus 'normally cycling women' are recruited for their studies, and, as we are assured, after 'informed consent' submit their bodies to invasive procedures (drug ingestion, frequent blood sampling with indwelling intravenous catheter, interference with diet and sleep, and repeated ultrasound and biopsy, etc.). In the name of science every possible phase of 'the subject's' menstrual cycle is probed and the specialist publications proudly illustrate the effects of RU 486 on the early follicular phase, the late follicular phase, the mid-luteal phase and the late luteal phase (see Stuenkel et al., 1990 for an overview and for a particularly harrowing study design).[14]

The literature often reveals diametrically opposed findings. The LH surge is delayed in some studies while in others it is normal; FSH levels are blocked, declined or are the same; hCG levels are significantly elevated (van Santen and Haspels, 1987: 436) or inhibited (Das and Catt, 1987: 600). Interpretations vary too, but without exception the papers reveal that RU 486 is poorly understood: 'The way in which mifepristone impairs corpus luteum function is unclear' (Nieman and Loriaux, 1988: 613); 'Whether this inhibition of gonadotropin [LH/FSH] release was a result of action at the hypothalamic and/or pituitary level is unknown' (Wolf et al., 1989: 185); 'The exact molecular mechanisms which mediate the negative effects of antihormones including RU 486 are not yet clear' (Ortmann et al., 1989: 295). Some findings suggest that in addition to its antiprogesterone activities, RU 486 has a progesterone-like (agonist) effect (Collins et al.,1986; Wolf et al., 1987; Parinaud et al., 1990). Other studies found that admin-istration of RU 486 without progesterone inhibited gonado-tropin secretion, and posit that RU 486 might have an independent – and unknown – mode of action in addition to its progesterone receptor blocking qualities (Wolf *et al.*, 1989: 189).[15] As Shi and Zhu put it:

> Early reports emphasized the local direct effect of RU 486 at the progesterone receptor level in the uterus ... However, the present study suggests that RU 486 and progesterone *compete* with one another at the levels of uterus, pituitary and hypothalamus, supporting the hypothesis that RU 486 interrupts early pregnancy and induces menses *by a multiple mode of action* (1990: 126; our emphasis).

RU 486 has also been tested as a menstrual inducer when administered before a missed period. However, when used to induce menstruation, the drug's failure rates are high, e.g. two out of eleven women had ongoing pregnancies (van Santen and Haspels, 1987). In another study which adminstered two doses of RU 486 to 12 women (the first on the day of the expected menses, the second eight days later), 22 pregnancies in 137 cycles (16%) occurred. (The unethical nature of this experiment is staggering!) The researchers concluded that 'because of the high failure rate, use of RU 486 ... cannot be advocated as a "once a month contraceptive"' (Couzinet *et al.*, 1990: 1039). These failure rates also rule out its acceptability as a morning-after pill. Moreover, because of its long and still undetermined half-life, it interferes with the next cycle, 'causing delay of follicular maturation and then disturbing periodicity' (Baulieu, 1988b: 127). In an experiment with RU 486 tampons used with monkeys, IVF researcher, Gary Hodgen,[16] states that 'After RU 486 administration, the next ovarian cycle and ovulation were often delayed, *sometimes for several weeks*' (1985: our emphasis). Baulieu himself suggests, '. . . one now needs a compound or an association of compounds acting for a relatively short time in order to avoid spill-over in the next ovulation' (*idem.*).

Some recent evidence suggests that RU 486 acts *directly*

on the ovary at the receptor level (Schreiber *et al.*, 1983; Di Mattina *et al.*, 1987), and impairs folliculogenesis. In some clinical trials, this manifests as a marked decline in E_2 (estradiol) levels (Shoupe *et al.*, 1987; Stuenkel *et al.*, 1990). In turn this delays – or inhibits – ovulation. A group of Finnish researchers posit that this characteristic of RU 486 is *reversible*. They also state that a subsequently administered synthetic progestin (e.g. NET, Primolut N) may lead to an estrogen-free oral contraceptive (Luukkainen *et al.*, 1988; Kekkonen *et al.*, 1990). Despite the fact that one of these studies – the Luukkainen *et al.* experiment – was restricted to *eight* women, and only two women had cycles without ovulation, these findings were picked up by the US *Ob. Gyn. News* under the headline 'RU 486 and Progestin Combination Could Yield Estrogen Free-OC [oral contraceptive]' (1989: 38).

In a later 1990 experiment with *seven* women, the same researchers noted, with surprise, some follicular growth during RU 486 administration (Kekkonen *et al.*, 1990).[17] Earlier trial findings by van Santen and Haspels in Holland (1987) showed that disturbances in a woman's cycle resulted from an egg of a delayed ovulation which later matured and in fact was fertilized 'inadvertently'. These two experiments make clear that the hailing of RU 486 as a new 'breakthrough in contraception' is thus far without foundation.

There is no evidence in the Luukkainen *et al.* study that they followed up on women's subsequent menstrual cycles. They state that, 'After termination of the RU 486 treatment, follicular development and luteinization occurred similarly as during the control cycle *in the majority of women*' (1988: 963). With *eight* women in their study, what was the majority of women and what happened to the others? If additionally RU 486 exerts a direct inhibitory intraovarian action by suppressing ovarian steroidogenesis [the production of estrogen (estradiol) and progesterone], the question must be asked whether and how this inhibition will affect the remaining thousands of immature eggs in a woman's ovary that were exposed to RU 486. In other words, a drug which in fact might have long-term effects on folliculogenesis, ovulation and hence future fertility is declared 'safe and effective', whereas, in reality, the mechanism(s) by which it might exert this action remain(s) unknown.

We are told, however, 'that RU 486 and two of its major metabolites can readily cross the blood follicle barrier of human pre-ovulatory follicles' (Cekan *et al.*, 1988: 131), a fact acknowledged by Baulieu in 1989b (p. 1353). This was established from an experiment on 21 'healthy female volunteers of proven fertility' who requested sterilization at the Department of Obstetrics and Gynaecology at the University of Aberdeen. Pre-treatment of the women involved ovulation induction with unacceptably high doses of clomiphene (150 mg for five days)[18] and hCG before they were administered a single dose of 100 mg RU 486. Thirty-four hours later, at laparoscopy, samples of blood and follicular fluid were collected. Both revealed high concentrations of RU 486 and two of its metabolites, more so in the follicular fluid than in the plasma.

In the same experiment, 48 'healthy' women requesting sterilization were first superovulated with clomiphene, and then received 100 mg of RU 486 before mature egg follicles were aspirated and fertilized *in vitro*. Fifty-six per cent of the eggs resulted in 'normal' fertilization (as compared with 66 per cent of those from a control group) and developed to the four to eight cell stage before they were frozen (Messinis and Templeton, 1988). The authors caution, however, that 'the developmental capacity of the oocytes after fertilization *in vitro* could not be fully determined, since the cleaving embryos were not replaced in a recipient uterus' (p. 594).[19] In contrast, another experiment regarding the effect of RU 486 on sperm-egg interaction in mice found that RU 486 *inhibited* fertilization *in vitro* in a dose dependent manner which could not be reversed by the addition of progesterone (Juneja and Dodson, 1990).[20]

Further questions arise from the observation by Shoupe *et al.* that the dominant follicle whose development was delayed by RU 486 may 'undergo spontaneous recovery' (1987: 1423). What will be the 'quality' of an egg that has undergone previous chemical arrest? If a woman *after* RU 486 decides to become pregnant, does she need to worry about RU 486 residues and/or irreversible damage to that follicle and perhaps others too? And what about cycle disturbances? To our knowledge no long-term follow-up studies of women after RU 486/PG have been undertaken to evaluate later pregnancies and menstrual cycles. The study of Régine Sitruk-Ware *et al.* is the only one we know of which includes a follow-up visit after three months (1990, RU 486 only). Sitruk-Ware *et al.* reported 'regular bleeding patterns' in 83 out of 99 women. (Twenty-five women did not reply.) However, because they put women on hormonal contraception, these are 'phantom' periods which are very different from periods due to the chain of hormonal events involved in a woman's 'natural' menstrual cycle. To call them 'regular bleeding' is a misrepresentation. Of even more concern is the fact that of the remaining 16 women, four experienced irregular bleeding and three had one episode of abnormal bleeding (three were pregnant again, one requested a further RU 486 termination; p. 234); the bleeding patterns of the remaining five women are missing. Sitruk-Ware also comments that one of the women initially considered a success had a curettage performed two months later because of abnormal bleeding. The curettage showed residual decidual material (1990: 234). It is alarming to think that such incomplete terminations might be quite frequent but will go undetected unless women return to their doctors because of bleeding episodes.

Finally, the questions must be asked, can RU 486 act *directly* on the fertilized egg/embryo and what is known about potential teratogenic effects. This is especially important because RU 486 induced abortion continues over a prolonged period, during which a number of women may change their mind and decide to *continue* the pregnancy.

In 1985, Frydman *et al.* wrote in *The Lancet* that their research on second-trimester pregnant women conclusively demonstrated that mifepristone crossed the placenta and that the absence of fetal toxicity was yet to be demonstrated (p. 1252). A year later, studies of cell cultures from seven to twelve-week-old embryos, which were obtained from conventional pregnancy termination (Bischof *et al.*, 1986), were compared with placentas obtained from normal deliveries and then immersed in RU 486 (Das and Catt, 1987). These studies demonstrated clearly that in early embryonic development RU 486 acts directly on the trophoblast which later grows into the placenta. In late stages of pregnancy, RU 486 inhibits the production and reduces the secretion of placental hormones. In both cases the researchers posit that this was due to inhibited production of hCG. There is limited and contradictory data on whether this direct action on the trophoblast/placenta might result in retardation of the embryos and contribute to the birth of children with abnormalities.

In their study designed to investigate the effect of RU 486 on embryo transport and preimplantation development in mice Y. Q. Yang and J. T. Wu administered RU 486 orally at 100mg/kg/day for two days to female mice, caged with male mice.[21] (Compared with the 600 mg commonly administered to women this represents roughly a tenfold increase.) The next day the mice were 'sacrificed', and oviducts and uteri removed and flushed for embryos. Compared with controls, the treated mice had fewer embryo numbers reaching the blastocyt stage (35 per cent versus 77 per cent) and generally fewer embryos. In addition, 69 per cent of the embryos were located in the oviducts. Yang and Wu conclude that 'RU 486 could retain the embryos in the oviduct but expel those having entered the uterus' (1990: 553). This finding is of great concern because it further indicates that RU 486 may cause ectopic pregnancies. The authors also state that the delay in implantation 'suggests strongly that estrogen secretion may be affected in some way' (*ibid.*). The results also showed 'that RU 486 could act *directly on the embryos causing a complete degeneration at high doses*' (*idem.*, our emphasis). Yang and Wu write that, 'The mechanism by which RU 486 acts directly on the embryo is not known at present'. In a personal communication to RK (May 1990), J. T. Wu commented that it was not established whether RU 486 worked on the pituitary or the hypothalamus and that 'we have no idea how RU 486 acts on the embryo'.

Yang and Wu are not alone in finding that RU 486 could have teratogenic effects on embryos. Jost reported fetal anomalies in rabbits from RU 486 treatment at sub-abortive dosage in 1986. On the other hand, Wolf *et al.* (including Roussel Uclaf researchers Dubois, Ulman and Baulieu) found no indication of teratogenicity, developmental abnormalities or differentials in survival or growth rates of monkey embryos exposed to RU 486. However, their numbers were small – limited in fact to the birth of a single 'normal' baby monkey after RU 486 administration. Another experiment with six RU 486 exposed fetuses within the same study resulted in only five 'normal' deliveries, the other being stillborn. The authors conclude that exposure to RU 486 during early stages of embryonic development 'is not likely to produce a high incidence of developmental lesions' (1990: 90). For us, nothing less than a zero incidence of developmental lesions is acceptable.

Likewise, findings from women who underwent RU 486/PG termination but then changed their minds and carried the pregnancy to term, are inconclusive. In 1988, the *British Medical Journal* noted one case where a French woman was reported to have given birth to a child with malformations (Dorozynsky, 1988: 1292). In a brief report in *Nature* (it is unclear whether this refers to the same French woman's abandoned RU 486 termination), an 18-

week fetus previously exposed to RU 486 was found to have 'a very severe oligoamnios [less than normal amniotic fluid]' (Henrion, 1989: 110). Given the potential risk of embryotoxicity, Henrion therefore strongly recommends that women are informed of the dangers, should they decide to continue the pregnancy following RU 486 exposure. This is why French women must sign a form that says they will agree to a conventional termination if RU 486/PG fails.

A report in *The Lancet* indicated normal development after exposure to mifepristone in early pregnancy (Lim *et al.*, 1990) with two women who delivered normal babies after RU 486 (but not PG) administration.[22] Based on these few accounts, there are no guarantees for a so-called 'normal' development of embryos exposed to RU 486. Follow-up is urgently needed on the considerable number of women documented in the RU 486 studies as 'being lost' in the process.

To summarize this introduction to RU 486 biology, many of the findings from research and clinical experiments are inconclusive and/or contradictory. It is therefore crucial to stress once more that neither endocrinology nor reproductive medicine has a concise understanding of the complex hormonal interactions that take place in a human female body. It is equally crucial to ask whether it is ethically and morally justifiable to once again use women as living test-sites for scientific manipulation and experimentation. In the case of RU 486/PG abortion these problems are compounded by the unknown interactions between *two* powerful drugs. In the following chapter we will investigate the nature and action of prostaglandins.

CHAPTER FOUR

The Role of Prostaglandins: Known and Unknown Dangers

Discussion of the abortion pill solely in terms of RU 486 is no longer possible. In what we see as a contrived protocol, RU 486 advocates now prescribe a prostaglandin (PG) medication, two to three days after the RU 486 pills have been swallowed, to reduce its abortion failures from 40 per cent to the present figure of five per cent. While PGs partly salvage the reputation of RU 486 as an 'effective' abortion pill, they subtract from any claim that RU 486 is 'safe'. PGs are by no means new to chemical abortion, having a dubious history that spans more than 20 years. As early as 1972, a Prostaglandin Task Force was established by the World Health Organization's (WHO) Expanded Programme of Research, Development and Research Training in Human Reproduction. The investigations of the Task Force were the initial, wide-scale venture into chemical abortion. Not unexpectedly, the agenda that justified the Task Force's existence, together with its funding, was population control via the application of PG to the post-conceptional regulation of fertility. Not unexpectedly either, it was women from various Asian countries who were the specified 'targets'.

The following sections contain information about PGs, first to acknowledge the complexities of these powerful substances which regulate the normal function of major body organs. A second section identifies some of the advantages and disadvantages of PG medications in health disorders that are of a non-gynecological and non-obstetrical nature. The third section examines the morals of those recommending PG approaches to pregnancy terminations and the grounds for rejecting these applications. In the second and third sections, some of the clinical limitations of PGs are discussed, with reference to hazards that have important implications for women contemplating chemical abortion. The fourth and final section comments on the PG/antiprogesterone abortion approach, comparing RU 486 with other antiprogesterones which have not been commercially marketed.

What Are Prostaglandins?

PGs belong to an important group of biochemical molecules that are collectively referred to as eicosanoids.[1] These molecules are not stored in any cell so that biosynthesis is limited by the availability of free precursor fatty acid. Arachidonic acid, together with its precursor substances linoleic and α-linolenic acids, is essential for the complete nutrition of many animal species, including humans, and these acids provide the raw material for eicosanoid manufacture. Enzymes are required for the conversion, or biosynthesis, of arachidonic acid to eicosanoids. These enzymes are present within virtually every mammalian cell, the one possible exception being the red blood cell. Knowledge of eicosanoid interactions is extensive at the biochemical level, but is relatively sparse at the level required to fully understand their role in human health and disease.

The biochemical activity of PGs differs from that of hormones in that their effects are chiefly directed at sites near where they are produced. PGs have a major influence on smooth muscle and platelets and their important action

81

sites include endocrine organs, the central nervous system, autonomic postganglionic nerve terminals, sensory nerve endings, adipose [fat] tissue and lymphocytes which are white blood cells that are central to the immune system. The PGE_1, E_2 and I_2 molecules have the capacity to induce suppression of immune responsiveness (Redgrave *et al.*, 1991a). More recently a PGE_1 analogue has been applied clinically, as an added medication to hinder the rejection of kidney transplants (Moran *et al.*, 1990).

Present day understanding of PGs conceives that these molecules are produced from a surge of enzymatic activity within the cell, following a specific stimulus. The resulting PG molecules transmit messages to other nearby cells, after which the PGs are rapidly inactivated. This is a vitally important mechanism to ensure that cellular exposure to naturally occurring (endogenous) PG molecules persists for only a brief time. Synthetic PG analogues, developed as an external (exogenous) source of PG for therapeutic purposes, have chemical characteristics which distinguish them from the body's naturally-occurring PGs. The most striking difference lies in their respective half-lives. For the synthetic PGs, the half-life may extend to 18 and even 24 hours, whereas the half-life of naturally occurring PGs may be a mere fraction of a second. The prolonged half-life, which is associated with improved stability, accounts for the successful application of pharmaceutical PG preparations to potentially debilitating, and even life-threatening, clinical disorders. However, it is the extended life of synthetic PGs which calls into question the ethics of PG-induced regulation of women's fertility. The biological threat of synthetic, stable PGs in pregnancy termination, which in itself is obviously not an illness, may be further amplified by the possible absence of nature's mechanism which inactivates naturally occurring PGs to ensure the body's brief exposure to these potent molecules. Additionally, the dosages of synthetic PGs, required to successfully terminate pregnancy, are extravagantly greater than that encountered by the body's individual cells in their natural environment. Therapeutic applications may be justified because they benefit patients whose continued existence, together with the quality of that existence, is jeopardized by an ongoing disease process. On the other hand, the advantages of PGs in these situations is not a licence for their application to healthy women seeking to terminate pregnancy.

Prostaglandins In the Treatment of Human Health Disorders

The understanding of the limits and safe usage of PG medications is in its infancy, but many of its clinical restrictions identify the potential risks for healthy women from a PG-containing chemical abortion 'cocktail'. PGs have been used, with favorable outcomes, in critical illnesses such as septic shock, adult respiratory stress syndrome, cardiac dysfunction, upper gastrointestinal haemorrhage, myocardial infarction, and liver and renal failure. One threatening long-term biological consequence of the PG component of the chemical abortion 'cocktail' is that most PG analogues inhibit the immune response. Misoprostol, a synthetic PGE_1 analogue, has been shown to reduce the incidence of rejection episodes in kidney transplant patients, while simultaneously protecting the kidney transplant from the toxic effects of other immunosuppressive drugs (Moran *et al.*, 1990).

Misoprostol is one of the few PG analogues that has oral bio-availability. It was recently reported (Altman, 1991) to be Baulieu's new PG additive, which he now advocates as a *simpler way to use the RU 486 abortion pill*, either unaware that it has little uterine effects and/or unconcerned with its immunosuppressive properties. Immune suppression in kidney, heart, liver and bone marrow transplant patients constitutes one of those ethical compromises, for while it is accompanied by an increased incidence of cancer and fatal infection, death from a terminal illness is the alternative to a successful transplant for these people. Proponents of PGs in pregnancy-related procedures claim that a single exposure to a *'small dose of prostaglandin'* has no effect on the immune system, but Di Francesco *et al.* (1990) have reported that isolated immune insults are more harmful than those of a chronic nature (as practised in transplantation).

We are unaware of any studies which assure healthy women that RU 486 and PG, *taken together*, does not weaken immune defence against malignancy and infection. Synthetic PG analogues, in microgram (abbreviated to mcg and one thousand times less than a milligram) amounts, induce sufficient immune suppression in animals to delay the rejection of experimental heart and kidney transplants (Wiederkehr *et al.*, 1990 and Redgrave *et al.*, 1991b). Gemeprost and sulprostone are both PGE_2 analogues, that are administered in milligram amounts (abbreviated to mg and one thousand times greater than a microgram) with RU 486 to induce abortion. Where gemeprost is administered as a vaginal pessary, as opposed to an intramuscular PG, the total amount is concentrated locally in the uterine region leading to levels far in excess of physiological concentrations. Until proven otherwise, women's exposure to synthetic PG during abortion procedures can be regarded as an immune insult.

Numerous clinical trials have compared the value of PG therapy in the healing of gastric and duodenal (stomach) ulcers. Sontag *et al.*, (1985) estimated the misoprostol duodenal ulcer healing rate in non-critically ill patients to be 64.9 per cent after treatment with 0.4 mg of misoprostol per day compared with 47.4 per cent in the placebo-treated group. Episodes of diarrhea occurred twice as frequently in the misoprostol group. Misoprostol trials, and those of Trimoprostil (a PGE_2), Rosaprostol (a prostanoic acid) and Enprostil (a dihydro-PGE_2), have failed to show a healing rate superior to that of cimetidine (Tagemet) which is probably the most frequently prescribed gastric ulcer medication. In fact, the numerical advantage has remained in favor of cimetidine and, since it is free of gastrointestinal side-effects, it remains the preferred gastric ulcer therapy. In contrast, the gastrointestinal side-effects of PGs in abortion procedures are trivialized, when diarrhea, superimposed on abortion's physical and psychological demands, is especially dehumanizing.

In healthy humans, the effect of both PGE_1 and PGE_2 is to increase the heart rate. Cardiovascular (heart and blood vessel) collapse has been observed following the obstetrical and gynecological use of PGs and is attributed to PG escaping into the blood stream which causes severe pulmonary hypertension and/or anaphylactic shock (an exaggerated and life-threatening allergic reaction). In anaesthetized pregnant women, PGs increase pulmonary resistance by 100 per cent and cause a three fold increase in work for the right side of the heart (Secher *et al.*, 1982). Even a minimal amount of PG, instilled intra-amniotically, can cause cardiovascular complications by leaking into the blood stream. Roussel Uclaf has expressed its concern for the cardiovascular hazards of synthetic PGs – no doubt reinforced by identical complications that caused the death of a 31-year-old woman in March, 1991 – and warns that RU 486/PG termination is contraindicated for women with history of cardiovascular-related conditions such as angina, cardiac arrhythmia, heart failure and high blood pressure.

Endogenous PGs have an important role in maintaining kidney function in patients with renal disease, so that medications which are PG-inhibitors, including many non-steroidal, anti-inflammatory drugs such as aspirin, can cause episodes of acute renal failure. Waltman *et al.*, (1973) recognized the importance of the PG-inhibiting property of certain medications in the context of abortion. They reported that women taking aspirin and indomethacin had a significantly delayed onset of abortion, compared with women receiving the same abortion treatment but not taking anti-inflammatory drugs. In relation to RU 486/PG-induced abortion, this means that many mild analgesics are inappropriate for counteracting the pain, as their use would further delay the onset of abortion and/or further increase the chemical abortion failure rate. This accounts for the prescription of opiate analgesics, pethidine for example, to counteract the pain from RU 486/PG treatment. We would suspect that women taking anti-inflammatory drugs, such as Indocin, Clinoril, Advil, Motrin or Naprosyn for arthritis-related inflammatory conditions, are at increased risk of incomplete abortion. Roussel Uclaf does not warn RU 486/PG consumers against the combined use of anti-inflammatory drugs and chemical abortion.

RU 486 proponents, especially those in the US, claim that chemical abortion progress is hindered by the absence of PG preparations that are appropriate for RU 486 salvage operations. This is viewed as a stumbling block to swift licensing of RU 486 and *'a small dose of prostaglandin'* by health authorities. G. D. Searle (USA) and Schering (Germany), which respectively manufacture Cytotec (misoprostol) and Nalador (sulprostone), have given us reason to understand that their products are *not* marketed for use with RU 486 in abortion procedures. Schering's comment of 19 March 1991 reads: 'We do not indicate the use of our product in combination with Mifepristone. Our information material on Nalador does not make any reference to such a combination' (pers. comm. to LD and RK).

Many assume that fear of moral backlash accounts for the reluctance of pharmaceutical companies to market PGs in forms suitable for abortion purpose. However, 'off-label' prescription of drugs is a frequent medical practice, once government approval has been obtained for a drug's specified ('on-label') use.[2] Thus, even if PGs are not licensed as abortifacients, this does not preclude their 'off-label' use with RU 486 in abortion procedures. Nalador and Cytotec are already two PGs which have been prescribed in this fashion, in the UK, France and Sweden, to terminate pregnancy with RU 486. We would contend, of course, that there simply would not be any PG requirement, were RU

486 the 'miracle pill' its supporters proclaim.

RU 486 advocates have capitalized on the inequitable standards operative in the management of women's reproductive health, to have women believe that *'RU 486 and a small dose of prostaglandin'* is a superior, safe and effective alternative to conventional abortion methods. The intention in the following section is to increase readers' perception of the importance of naturally-occurring PGs in reproductive health, with a view to establishing an 'informed' resistance to the continuing abuse of women's bodies in pregnancy-related procedures.

The Role and Application of Prostaglandins in Obstetrics and Gynecology

PGs were initially discovered in human semen, where they are probably regulated by progesterone to influence sperm and egg transport. PGE levels within seminal fluid may be important in male fertility, and, due to their immunosuppressive properties, may act to protect the sperm component of the fertilized ovum from immune attack that would result in its destruction at or before the time of its uterine implantation.

Contrary to their limited influence on male reproduction, PGs play a pivotal role in the regulation of women's reproductive biology. Abnormalities in natural PG production are associated with a number of gynecological and obstetrical disorders, including primary dysmenorrhea (menstrual cramps). Events which are PG dependent are cervical softening in the final stages of pregnancy, and (independent of pregnancy) uterine contractions, the initiation of ovarian follicular growth and rupture, egg cell maturation, and corpus luteum formation and rupture. Though ovarian processes are chiefly regulated by hormones, the hormone effects are probably modulated by PGs.[3]

Obstetrical and gynecological use of PGs commenced in

the early 1970s when oral, intravenous and local PG preparations were used instead of oxytocin as a means of cervical ripening for the induction of both labor and abortion. The following medical reports of PG applications identify the trivialization and disregard for issues that are of vital concern to women in the management of their reproductive health. The examples cited are in no way selective, and represent only a small part of an enormous body of medical literature.

Euler *et al.* (1989), investigated the effects of Arbaprostil, a PGE_2 analogue, on the uterus of women who were not pregnant and others who were. The purpose of the study was to avoid litigation as a result of the abortifacient activity of the PG when administered at anti-ulcer dosages. Changes in intra-uterine pressure indicated that single doses of Arbaprostil caused no significant effects on uterine muscle tone in women who were not pregnant, nor in first trimester pregnant women. Assured that single dose Arbaprostil had no abortion-inducing potential, multiple dose studies were then undertaken with up to eight times the maximal amount intended for gastrointestinal therapy. Abortion rates increased from zero per cent to nine per cent in a dose-dependent manner, as did the gastrointestinal side-effects of nausea, vomiting and diarrhea. The incidence of diarrhea was 38 per cent from 400 mcg (0.4 mg) of Arbaprostil and 70 per cent from 1,600 mcg or 1.6 mg of Arbaprostil. These figures probably influenced Euler *et al.* to issue the following condemnation of the PG usage in abortion procedures (1989: 97):

> At doses where we encountered minimal uterine effects manifested, primarily by vaginal spotting, the incidence of gastrointestinal side effects was already very high. If the absolute dose or frequency of administration were increased further, one can confidently predict that the gastrointestinal side effects would become intolerable to the patients as has been previously documented when PGE_2 or its synthetic derivatives have been given orally or intramuscularly.

Intolerable? Certainly, women experiencing the adverse effects of PGs in abortion procedures have not received the same considerations.

Fetal distress can occur in high-risk pregnancies following the increased frequency of uterine contractions after labor induction with extra-amniotic PG. A number of reports even cite fetal death in utero. Quinn and Murphy (1981) reported two $PGF_{2\alpha}$-related fetal deaths and suggested that continuous monitoring of fetal heart rate and uterine contractions of all women with high-risk pregnancies was necessary during delivery, if they had been administered local PGs for cervical softening.

A case study reported by Simmons and Savage (1984), attributed a neonatal death, following the premature separation of a normally situated placenta, to the induction of labor with a 3 mg PGE_2 pessary. After the death, these investigators administered smaller PG doses to women whose cervices softened more spontaneously and no similar incidents were observed. This report indicated that the potential dangers of PG usage were increased by three factors: the mistaken perception of 'simple' labor induction with PG methods, inadequate assessment of women during pregnancy and an unwillingness to publish these adverse incidents in the appropriate medical journals.

An additional fetal hazard of PGs in obstetrics and gynecology is the possibility that these drugs induce teratogenesis (malformation in embryonic/fetal development; see misoprostol later in this chapter). *'RU 486 and a small dose of prostaglandin'* fails to induce abortion in one woman of every 20 and, as a result, any continuing pregnancy has an increased risk of fetal abnormality. Fetal hydrocephalus and abnormal growth was reported by Wood *et al.* (1987), following an unsuccessful second trimester abortion attempt with oxytocin and PGE_2. The woman later gave birth, in her 37th week of pregnancy, to a female child, who had epilepsy, severely retarded development, severe vision impairment and spastic quadriplegia, all attributed

89

to the PG exposure during fetal development. Information on PG teratogenesis, although sparse, does support the widespread assumption that a fetus exposed to these chemicals will be deprived of oxygen. Another clinical report (Collins and Mahoney, 1983) described hydrocephalus and abnormal toes and fingers in a pregnancy that continued after a failed abortion attempt with $PGF_{2\alpha}$ during the first trimester. To our knowledge there are no studies to establish whether the teratogenic risk from PG exposure may be even greater when the pregnancy continues following exposure to both RU 486 and PG.

Women, too, are at risk from PG-induced cervical softening for labor or pregnancy termination, although there are conflicting opinions over the degree of risk. Husslein et al. (1989) described the use of PG in tubal pregnancy terminations as 'highly encouraging'. However, Dietl and Lippert (1990), responded that 'the associated burden and dangers for the patient were given little consideration' (p. 707), and expressed specific concerns about the complications due to intra-uterine $PGF_{2\alpha}$ which may injure, or, in some cases, kill women.

At least eight women have died following the use of $PGF_{2\alpha}$ in legal abortions performed in the US (Cates et al., 1977; Cates and Jordaan, 1979). Neither of the two women described in the 1979 report had any prior history of cardiac or neurological disorder. In fact, a *normal* electrocardiogram and electroencephalogram had been observed for one of the women. As such, this woman's case history serves to warn that screening for conditions that predispose to sudden collapse from PG may be of little value in predicting a fatal outcome. This particular woman, aged 26 years, collapsed three minutes after an intra-amniotic PG-induced abortion procedure at a university teaching hospital. Despite the immediate and elaborate resuscitation measures instantly available, her death could not be averted. She aborted six days after the instillation procedure but remained in a coma until her death about four weeks later.

Although deaths are rare, two of the American women experienced a number of features observed in four other women who had serious, though non-fatal, complications during PG-induced termination procedures at a Scandinavian Clinic (Lange, 1983). The first of these four women experienced anaphylactic shock, 10 seconds after a $PGF_{2\alpha}$ instillation that resulted in breathing difficulties, violent nausea, stomach pains, slowing of the heart beat (bradycardia), and universal skin redness. This woman recovered without further complication. Two of the four women experienced anaphylactic shock, one immediately following $PGF_{2\alpha}$ (40 mg) instillation and the other 30 minutes after $PGF_{2\alpha}$ instillation. The fourth woman was less fortunate. She experienced nausea and vomiting immediately after a 40 mg $PGF_{2\alpha}$ instillation, developed bradycardia and severe bronchospasm before her heartbeat and breathing stopped. She was resuscitated, with restoration of normal cardiac activity within 30 minutes, but to the report's date, retained an abnormal electro-encephalogram and was demented due to deprivation of the brain's oxygen supply (cerebral anoxia).

Because violent stomach pain, vomiting and diarrhea are known effects of PGs, Lange (1983) suggested that PG-induced complications were due to the leakage of $PGF_{2\alpha}$ into the women's circulation. So, too, are the triggering of breathing difficulties and epileptic seizures, but the most serious effects are slowing heartbeat and low blood pressure which may lead to cardiac arrest.

Cervical injury is described by Kajanoja (1983) as a severe complication of PG-induced termination that can interfere with 'future reproductive performance'. In his series of 510 intra-amniotic $PGF_{2\alpha}$-induced abortions, nine women (1.8 per cent) suffered a cervical tear. This injury was more than twice as frequent (4.1 per cent) in women who were pregnant for the first time. PG-instillation has resulted in perforation extending from the cervix to the vagina. Ingvardsen and Eriksen (1979) reported that a rupture of this type was associated with a persistent cervico-vaginal fistula (a passage between the cervix and vagina created by injury). In one woman, vaginal 16,16-dimethyl PGF_2 caused a rupture of her womb during pregnancy termination. The fetus and placenta were later found within her abdomen (Jerve *et al.*, 1979). Cervical tears are more frequent when PGs are administered via the intra-amniotic route, but they also occur as a result of extra-amniotic, intramuscular and vaginal PG. In this context, sulprostone (intramuscular PG) and gemeprost (vaginal PG) may salvage the RU 486 reputation as an 'effective' abortion pill but at what price? The inheritance may be a torn cervix, a ripped vagina and/or chronic discomfort from an additional connecting channel (fistula) between the cervix and vagina.

The first clinical report of PG-induced abortion involved the intravenous infusion of $PGF_{2\alpha}$ (Karim and Filshie, 1970). A year later, Csapo *et al.* commented, perhaps aware of the prolonged trauma experienced by women subjected to the procedure and the excessive PG concentrations that the women were exposed to, that intravenous $PGF_{2\alpha}$ was not a recommendable method for inducing abortion (1971: 1059):

The use of an identical protocol (Upjohn* 002), employed in two recent studies and the present report yielded comparable results. In these trials, a total of 30 mid-trimester patients (12 to 16 weeks pregnant, excepting 3 first-trimester cases) were infused intravenously with *up to 200μ per minute of $PGF_{2\alpha}$ during a period of 12 hr. When this first treatment failed to induce abortion, the treatment was repeated the following day.* Only 23 per cent of the study patients aborted completely, 50 per cent had incomplete abortions and 27 per cent failed to abort. *Thus, 77 per cent of the combined group required surgical completion of $PGF_{2\alpha}$-induced abortion, and the majority experienced diarrhea, vomiting and nausea* (our emphasis).

Nonetheless Csapo *et al.* (1972) persisted with this new abortion approach since:

> As a consequence of deficiencies such as these, investigators have been *challenged to improve the clinical efficacy and acceptability* of $PGF_{2\alpha}$ treatment, either by altering the route of administration to allow a reduction in dosage or by using prostaglandins of greater efficacy (pp. 1059–60, our emphasis)

and implied that the 'in press' PG studies of Arpad Csapo would provide a concise understanding of the important mechanisms of chemically induced abortion to avoid its negative elements (p. 1062).

By 1972, the WHO Prostaglandin Task Force focused its chemical abortion program on the $PGF_{2\alpha}$ and PGE_2 analogues, despite their abysmal abortion failure rates (WHO, 1972). Many of the factors[4] which determine the abortion success rate of PGs were identified subsequent to the program's commencement, so that – like the current RU 486 promotion – it was a premature exercise. Here too, lies a further parallel, the general trend to acknowledge Bygdeman as the theorist responsible for the PG abortion approach, just as there is to acknowledge Baulieu with the anti-progesterone approach, when in truth it was the theories of Csapo *et al.*, which gave the impetus to both PG and RU 486-induced abortion. We condemn the practice of PG-induced terminations and oppose PG usage with, or without, RU 486.

Based on the following statement we would have thought that the WHO Scientific Group on Advances in Methods of Fertility Regulation was aware of the advantage of conventional abortion methods: 'It is evident that suction curettage is the method of choice for termination of pregnancy in the first 12 weeks of gestation. The method is associated with a surprisingly low incidence of complications as indicated by results from e.g. Eastern Europe' (1972:

92). WHO's motive for discarding the conventional approach to abortion was unclear. Particularly when at least one further important reservation had emerged from the PG approach: 'pregnancy termination by intra-amniotic PG cases beyond the 22nd week was probably not recommendable, as the foetus may sometimes survive the procedure' (*idem.*).

Irrespective of motive, WHO trials proceeded, unconcerned that physiological PG levels were dramatically increased by an experimental 25 mg amount of exogenous PG, albeit administered via the intra-amniotic route. Normally, in women these levels are in the nanogram or even pikogram range (a nanogram [abbreviated to ng] being 0.001 mcg, and a pikogram [abbreviated to pk] being 0.000001 mcg). This 25 mg dose, is the equivalent of 25,000 mcg or 25,000,000 ng of PG and requires a 2.5 million-fold dilution by body fluids or chemical decay before physiological levels are restored within the cervical region of women subjected to this amount of PG. The biological consequences of outrageously excessive PG concentrations, which may be further amplified by the use of stable, synthetic PG analogues, is unknown.

More recent PG-induced abortion procedures employ intra-amniotic, intramuscular or intra-vaginal delivery of the PG derivatives. The PGE_2 analogues, Cervagem (gemeprost) and Nalador (sulprostone) are those most frequently prescribed, gemeprost being a 1 mg vaginal pessary and sulprostone a 0.25 or 0.5 mg intramuscular injection. A 1982 symposium on Cervagem 'A New Prostaglandin in Obstetrics and Gynaecology', valorized Sultan M. M. Karim as 'the father, if not the grandfather, of PGs in the field of obstetrics'. Karim (1983), in his report to the symposium audience, listed the applications of exogenous PGs in gynecology and obstetrics that he judged to be the mimicry of natural processes:

> ...menstrual induction/termination of very early pregnancy, termination of first trimester pregnancy, pre-evacuation

cervical dilation in first trimester of pregnancy, termination of abnormal intra-uterine pregnancy, pre-induction cervical ripening, induction of labour, control of post-partum haemorrhage, and post-partum and post-surgical retention of urine (pp. 15–16).

We would seriously question how many of these applications are actually in women's best interests.

It was acknowledged during this symposium that PG-induced termination of first trimester pregnancy compared *unfavorably* with vacuum aspiration on all accounts (except that it eliminated the need to mechanically dilate the cervix). Vacuum aspiration, on the other hand, can be performed within minutes, at an outpatient clinic, is complete in 99 per cent of women and has minimal immediate or long-term side effects, whereas PG-induced abortion takes several hours, requires overnight hospitalization, is incomplete in more than 50 per cent of women (vacuum aspiration or curettage are then necessary), with most women experiencing uterine cramps, vomiting and diarrhea.

At the same Cervagem symposium, Marc Bygdeman, a member of the WHO Prostaglandin Task Force, presented details of his experiences with PGs in obstetrics and gynecology. Three groups of women received alternative PG treatment to terminate first trimester pregnancies. One of the groups consisted of women, whose history included at least one previous pregnancy, who 'agreed to treat themselves at home'. This parallels the fashion in which RU 486 is presented as a 'take-home' package while retaining the sequential nature of multiple medical visits. As Bygdeman *et al.* elaborated (1983: 64–65):

Three visits, the first to confirm pregnancy and receive treatment under medical supervision (except for *those women who agreed to treat themselves at home*), a second for the estimation of haemoglobin, plasma ß-hCG, and a third for gynaecological examination, further haemoglobin and ß-hCG estimations, which were used for a preliminary judgement of complete abortion, incomplete abortion, or non-interrupted pregnancy and, if the state of the pregnancy was not obvious, then an ultrasound examination (our emphasis).

Besides the inherent dangers from medically unsupervised PG administration, the idea of take-home-PG passes responsibility for its preservation over to women. This has been ignored in the debate of RU 486-based abortion. Especially in developing countries, women are unlikely to have refrigeration facilities in their homes. Nor do they have access to rapid transportation to obtain appropriately preserved medications from medical centers. No doubt, women will be blamed for unsuccessful chemical abortions, where their failure to adequately preserve the PG can be heaped on to their other 'misdemeanours', such as cigarette smoking and alcohol consumption.

Bygdeman claimed that the PG success rate was similar to that obtained with vacuum aspiration and that treatment failure was rare. Not unexpectedly, he did not supply figures to support the claim that vacuum aspiration or suction curettage had the same six per cent to eight per cent failure rate as the PG method. Nor did he provide any criteria to justify the trivialization of such frequent failures as 'rare events'. The incidence of gastrointestinal side effects was similar in all three treatment groups, where 40–50 per cent of women experienced vomiting and diarrhea. Bygdeman chose to phrase the negative as positive, thereby trivializing this frequency of gastrointestinal side effects: 'Between 50 per cent and 60 per cent of patients experienced *no* vomiting or diarrhea. The percentage of patients with four or more episodes of both symptoms together was 6 per cent or less. . .' (Bygdeman *et al.*, 1983: 67). He concluded that PG treatment offered a safe, effective means of pregnancy termination.

The side-effects and dangers of PG-induced abortions have been acknowledged by some within the medical profession, even though that recognition may have been more from a perspective of protecting the profession, rather than genuine care for women. Kajanoja (1983), in a review of PG-induced second trimester pregnancies, warned of the stressful nature of the procedure and the possible repercussions if improvements were not forthcoming (p. 145):

> I have observed that inductions lasting more than one day and night are very distressing, and should be regarded as failures . . . The severity of the side-effects varies from patient to patient. In some women they are very distressing, and certainly limit the use of prostaglandins. If it is intended to administer PGs to a woman, she should be informed of the advantages and disadvantages. Otherwise, we in the Nordic countries might find ourselves in the same situation as the Federal Republic of Germany, where a women's movement has been formed against PGs, the doctors who use them and the pharmaceutical companies who produce them. . .

Nowhere in the current discussion about chemical abortion is it mentioned that this is a case of 'déjà vu'. In the late 70s, chemical abortion with the PG sulprostone was introduced for first trimester abortion and hailed by gynecologists as a 'safer' abortion method. Especially in Germany, many hospitals advocated it as the *sole* method to terminate first trimester pregnancies: an argument strikingly similar to the current promotion of RU 486/PG by some of its proponents.

However, PG abortion met with considerable resistance. The feminist health movement protested sharply against its introduction in Germany and Switzerland (e.g. *Les Frondeuses*, 1979: 3–4). With the slogan 'For Humane Abortion – Against Prostaglandins', health activists from Berlin and Hamburg exposed it as a form of *medical violence* against women during a tribunal against the § 218 (the German abortion §) in 1980 (Gruppe Prostaglandine, 1981: 3).

A year earlier, in 1979, two feminist lawyers had already launched a law suit against a local hospital on behalf of a woman who had become very ill and suffered extreme pains during PG administration for a first trimester abortion. She had not been told about adverse effects and was never asked her permission to submit to this experimental method that had not yet been approved as a treatment (*Courage*, 1979: 10–11). The law suit led to an investigation of the hospital and it was found that doctors had used PG on 400 women for first trimester abortion without informing them about the experimental status of Nalador (sulprostone) or its adverse effects. Four doctors pleaded guilty of using a non-approved drug and had to pay fines. The woman's law suit, however, was dropped and she did not receive any compensation. Similarly, a law suit against Schering (Nalador's manufacturer) was abandoned. The drug company claimed that they did not require written consent for the trials as this would deny their trust in doctors' ethics to inform their patients of the nature of the experiment. *Furthermore, it would violate the doctors' confidentiality.* In addition, they argued that the trials with Nalador had been done on *ill* people where oral consent was all that was necessary, thus categorizing pregnancy as disease (Gruppe Prostaglandine, 1981: 40–41).

The debate in Germany took on such dimensions with women protesting against PGs by sending lists of signatures to the German Ministry of Health, writing critical articles and organizing workshops to discuss the procedure and its adverse effects, that in 1980, the Ministry of Health held official Hearings on PGs in Berlin. However, feminist health activists reported the event as, 'It was just a show. Each gynecologist praised his research results – no proof necessary – and comparisons with alternative abortion methods were not sought' (*ibid.*: 4). This, too, strikes a familiar chord with the current debate about the 'second wave' of chemical abortion! 'Women who had used the PG method and described their negative experiences were silenced and labelled incompetent' (*idem.*). Nalador was deemed a suitable abortion method by the Ministry of Health and its use in Germany (and Switzerland) continued.

In an angry response, the women from Gruppe Prostaglandine in Hamburg published a 47-page documentation on PGs and their role in abortion in the hope that 'public pressure and the refusal by women to abort with PG will contribute to its prohibition' (*ibid.*: 43). Unfortunately, more than ten years later, PG abortion is still widespread in Switzerland and Germany, mainly in University Hospitals. Because of the many parallels to the current PG/RU 486 debate, we will briefly summarize the harrowing experience of a woman from the German documentation.

After admission for a first trimester termination A. is informed by a doctor that, at this hospital, all pregnancies – independent of age – are terminated by PG administration. Knowing about the long duration and pain involved A. is not happy with this news. But the doctor is very reassuring: from a medical point of view this method is much to be preferred over all other methods which are dangerous and lead to injuries. He is especially adamant about out-patient abortions and calls them 'irresponsible'. PG termination, he says, is really not too bad. Some women would expel the embryo after the first injection, others needed a second injection five hours later. So the maximum expected duration of the procedure would be ten hours and was 'really bearable'. The next day a D and C would be performed under general anaesthetic, which of course was totally without danger as the cervix was already softened.

A. doesn't like this information but can't reach her own physician who does out-patient abortions (he is on holidays). Another hospital puts her off for a few days...and she cannot bear to go through examinations and consultations with two doctors and a social worker again in order to gain approval for a legal termination. She agrees to PG termination.

A. receives the first injection and soon after feels dizzy and hot, and has mild cramping. Three hours later she starts bleeding, the cramps are more painful and she breaks out in sweats. A further hour later the pain has reached her tolerance threshold and she feels very nauseous. Half an hour later the pain has lessened somewhat but she is extremely cold. Five hours after the first injection the nurse appears with the second. A. protests, after all she has already had some bleeding, is it really necessary? The physician is called and decides that a second injection is indeed needed.

Immediately after this injection A. starts vomiting. She begins to shake uncontrollably and the pain becomes unbearable. Her feet and hands go numb, then her arms and her face. Her breathing becomes cramped, she wants to die. The other women in her room fetch the doctor and the nurse. Gradually the constricted breathing lessens. The pain is still unbearable, she still wants to die. But, she is told, she'll get a painkiller only later in order not to restrict the contractions. Three hours after the second injection, she starts expelling. But despite repeated attempts only a small amount of tissue is expelled. Gradually the pains lessen and she is given a sleeping tablet. Totally exhausted she falls asleep. More than ten hours have elapsed since the first injection.

The following morning A. receives a tranquilizing injection. In the afternoon a D and C is performed under general anaesthesia. The next day, still in hospital, a follow-up exam takes place. A. is totally exhausted and it takes her more than a week to recover. 'Each time', she says,

> when I talk with women who had an out-patient abortion, I feel this incredible anger surface. PG termination – especially up to the 12th week – is a totally unacceptable method against which we must strongly object. We must demand that at last hospitals too perform gentle out-patient suction terminations with a local anaesthetic (*ibid.*; summary in trans. by RK: 12–16).

Summarizing their case against PG abortion, the authors of the German documentation state that PG abortion serves *doctors*, not women, and that, 'the irresponsibility of most doctors against women goes hand in hand with their incapability and unwillingness to learn the suction method' (*ibid*: 42–43). We think this comment is equally pertinent today: instead of favoring a dubious chemical procedure, abortion providers who want to act in women's best interest should, instead, devote time and energy to train (lay) people to administer out-patient abortions (see Conclusion). Also, then and now, we protest against a method that is extremely painful and psychologically demanding: 10 hours of pain and fear, with a D and C the following day (under general anaesthesia) with the PG method and with RU 486/PG, up to two weeks of pain and doubt, followed possibly by a suction termination. The parallel reeks of women being made to suffer for demanding a termination which is a 'punishment' we strongly resent.

The continued practice of PG abortion has paved the way for RU 486 procedures in the 1990s. As a consequence, women now seeking abortion services are at increased threat, not simply from PGs, but from an RU 486-based chemical 'cocktail' that has unknown short- and long-term biological consequences from two second-rate chemicals.

Cameron and Baird (1984) compared the use of a 1 mg PGE_2 vaginal pessary (gemeprost) with extra-amniotic PGE_2 (prostin) in terminating early second trimester pregnancy. Gemeprost was placed in the vagina, and repeated every three hours until the products of conception were expelled, or until the frequency or severity of any side effects became so great as to warrant cessation of therapy, or until a total of five pessaries had been given. Prostin was administered at a constant rate of 0.1 mcg/hour until abortion occurred, to a maximum of 24 hours. As one has come to anticipate, women with a somewhat unusual pregnancy (called 'abnormal') or spontaneous abortion were excluded from the study, as were women with cardiovascular or pulmonary disease, allergy or epilepsy. Complete abortion rates were stated to be 77 per cent and 79 per cent from the respective treatments. The time between PG administration and abortion occurrence were similar for both groups, 839 minutes (14 hours!) in the vaginal pessary group and 897 minutes (15 hours!) in the extra-amniotic infusion group. However, these figures, on top of being scandalous, are a gross underestimate, since the 20 per cent of women who aborted outside of 24 hours were excluded from the analysis. Analgesic requirements were significantly different for women in the two groups, with those in the infusion group requiring pethidine injections twice as frequently as those in the pessary group. Side effects in the pessary versus the infusion group were: temperature higher than 37°C, 77 per cent versus 55 per cent; vomiting, 19 per cent versus 24 per cent; diarrhea, 12 per cent versus three per cent. According to Cameron and Baird (1984), no serious cardiovascular effects were seen, but hypotension occurred in 19 per cent of the pessary group and nine per cent of the infusion. (Hypotension is a known PG side-effect that may precede cardiac arrest). Again, according to Cameron and Baird, no excessive blood loss was encountered in either group of their experiment, yet one woman in the infusion group was transfused with five units of packed cells (this being the equivalent of five pints, or measured metrically, two liters of blood). Surgical terminations under general anaesthesia were performed in three women (two from the pessary group, and one from the infusion group) who did not abort successfully. This of course disregards the 20-odd per cent of women in each group who are obliterated from the records because they aborted outside of 24 hours. Furthermore, all women underwent an uterine evacuation after PG treatment, whether the abortion was complete or not. In retrospect, complete abortion, defined as the passage of the fetus and the placenta in its entirety, only occurred in 20 per cent of women in each group which contradicted the preliminary estimates of 77 per cent and 79 per cent abortion success rates. Despite these shortcomings, the pessary method was deemed highly acceptable to both 'patients and staff alike' (p. 1139). Considering that all women were subjected to a double abortion procedure, we were in no way surprised to learn that follow-up attendance was 'disappointing': less than 50 per cent of women from each treatment group!

Hill and McKenzie (1990) compared PG-induced termination of early pregnancy with conventional abortion methods, although this UK study was more due to the emerging interest in the now-dominant antiprogesterone approach, than in demonstrating PG superiority or inferiority. Results from PG terminations were compared with those obtained with suction aspiration under local anaesthesia during the same 10 year period. Suction aspiration is not, however, the most frequently used abortion method in the UK, with almost a third of terminations performed at less than eight weeks' gestation, usually by cervical dilatation and surgical evacuation of the uterus under general anaesthesia. Consequently the number of women whose abortions were induced by suction aspiration comprised only 265 whereas 865 women were managed with PGs. The side effects and transfusion rate were lower after aspiration (0.4 per cent and zero per cent) than from PG treatment (59 per cent and 1.3 per cent). An additional disadvantage of the PG treatment was that 8.5 per cent of women were readmitted for evacuation, whereas readmission was required of only 0.9 per cent of women after aspiration. The outcome, in terms of abortion rate and side effects, is an appalling indictment of PG-induced abortion.

A WHO (1987) multicenter study (termed 'trial') compared sulprostone with vacuum aspiration to terminate pregnancy (termed 'menstrual regulation'). Altogether 486 women, with 'admission criteria' of amenorrhea less than 49 days and 'normal general and gynaecological history and examination and giving informed consent that either a surgical or a medical treatment was to be used to induce "menstruation"' (pp. 950–951), were included in the randomized experiment. All women were hospitalized for at least eight hours, for either intramuscular injections of sulprostone at a dose of 0.5 mg, three times at three-hourly intervals, or vacuum aspiration that was usually performed under local anaesthetic. The protocol included recording of vital signs and body temperature at regular intervals, time of bleeding onset, uterine pain and side-effects, together with three follow-up visits at one, two and six to eight weeks post treatment. Intervention before the second follow-up visit was not permitted unless clinically indicated, e.g. for heavy bleeding, and the outcomes in these women were judged as incomplete abortions. Where women were still pregnant at the second follow-up visit, the pregnancy was terminated by vacuum aspiration. If the outcome remained in doubt at this visit, assessment was delayed until the third follow-up visit, and if curettage was necessary from the second follow-up visit to the first menstruation then the outcome was determined on the basis of histological examination. Where products of conception remained and were subsequently detected in the curettings, the outcome was classified as incomplete abortion. WHO concluded that sulprostone and vacuum aspiration were equally effective in terminating early pregnancy, the respective abortion rates being 91.1 per cent and 94.0 per cent. The figures for incomplete abortion and pregnancy continuation were 7.4 per cent and 1.5 per cent for the sulprostone-treated women, and 2.8 per cent and 3.2 per cent for the women who underwent vacuum-aspiration. Vomiting occurred in 29.6 per cent of sulprostone-treated women, diarrhea in 21.2 per cent and pain that necessitated analgesia via injection in 12.3 per cent. In contrast, the incidence of diarrhea, vomiting and analgesic requirement were merely 1.9 per cent, 0.0 per cent and 0.5 per cent in women who underwent vacuum aspiration. These abysmal figures, together with the extent of medical supervision and monitoring involved in the sulprostone protocol and its inherent danger as an abortion medication, are clear indications that the chemical abortion approach is inferior to conventional methods and is therefore eminently unacceptable.

A subsequent multicenter experiment (WHO, 1989b) investigated the effectiveness of a lower dose of sulprostone (0.25 mg) administered at four-hourly intervals, but made no comparison between sulprostone and vacuum aspiration effectiveness. An interim analysis indicated this protocol was clinically unacceptable, its abortion rate being only 41 per cent. The dose was therefore increased to the 0.5 mg level of the earlier experiment (WHO, 1987) and administered twice with a four-hourly interval between intramuscular injections. This, too, resulted in an unacceptable abortion rate, 67 per cent, and it was concluded that the sulprostone dose of the previous WHO study of 1987, three doses of 0.5 mg, represented the minimum dose for 'menstrual regulation'. In an interview with one of us (RK) in March 1991, Paul van Look of WHO, Geneva, indicated that a recently completed trial had shown that 0.25 mg of sulprostone was sufficient for RU 486/PG abortion. A month later, the French Ministry of Health advised that RU 486 should not be used with greater than 0.125 mg of sulprostone. This is a classic example of trial-and-error experimentation based on the unacceptable principle that near enough is good enough. (In addition, the reduction from 0.25 to 0.125 mg of sulprostone is meaningless, since it still requires a 100,000 fold dilution to become compatible with physiological levels.)

All of the PG experiments that we have chronicled in this chapter indicate no advantage for women from PG-based abortions. As discussed in Chapters Two and Three, nor has RU 486. It is irrational to expect that two chemicals, which have independently failed as abortifacients, will be miraculously transformed by their combination to become the successful and acceptable abortion method of the future. We posit that there is no chemical, least of all the

RU 486/PG-containing chemical cocktail, which is a viable alternative to conventional abortion. Moreover, RU 486 may not even be the best antiprogesterone developed to date, which is discussed in the final section of this chapter.

Prostaglandin/Antiprogesterone-induced Abortion

It was in fact Csapo, not Baulieu, as we are often led to believe, who first proposed the theory that blocking progesterone would terminate pregnancy (see also Chapter Three). He recognized that progesterone was vital to maintain the viability of an embryo implanted in the uterus (Csapo *et al.*, 1973). Pharmaceutical companies subsequently responded to this concept with research and development programs that identified at least four agents with antiprogesterone activity, epostane, RU 486 and two ZK analogues. Each has been proven to interrupt pregnancy in animal species such as rats, guinea pigs, sub-human primates and humans.

Experiments have identified unique chemical differences between these antiprogesterones, which account for varying activities in different animal species, and the pregnancy-stage at which their action is effective. Elger *et al.* (1987) compared the anti-fertility activity of RU 486 and the ZK analogues, 98.299 (onapristone) and 98.734 in the guinea pig[5] to demonstrate differences in their respective activities. The three drugs induced abortion in advanced pregnancy, but RU 486, even at the very high dose of 30.0 mg/day administered subcutaneously, failed to induce expulsions in more than 50 per cent of animals. In contrast, ZK 98.734 showed dose-dependent effects, was faster acting than RU 486, and at a dosage of 30.0 mg/day induced abortion in 100 per cent of animals. A quantitative assessment of myometrial PG sensitivity established the optimum duration of RU 486 or ZK-priming, with onapristone having significantly greater effectiveness than ZK 98.734 and RU 486 in elevating the myometrial sensitivity to subsequent administration of sulprostone or oxytocin.

In contrast to Baulieu who posited that RU 486 stimulated the production of endogenous uterine PGs, the studies of Elger *et al.*, (1987) indicated that there is no pre-existing 'intrinsic uterine stimulant', nor sufficient activation of uterine PG to induce the uterine contractions that ensure the expulsion of the fetus, following anti-progesterone-induced termination of pregnancy. Instead, RU 486 and other antiprogesterone analogues may create a PG deficit that persists for several days, and which serves to restrict abortion efficiency. Theoretically, *'the small dose of prostaglandin'*, which supplements RU 486 in abortion procedures, is a rescue medication to correct Baulieu's (and other promoters of the abortion pill) conceptual misunderstanding of antiprogesterone mechanisms. At the practical level, it is *'the small dose of prostaglandin'*, not RU 486, which is the dominant drug responsible for the expulsion of embryonic tissue after pregnancy interruption. Suppression of endogenous uterine PG production by antiprogesterone medications would imply that the expulsion of fetal tissue, which occurs in 60–80 per cent of women undergoing RU 486-induced abortion without PG, was merely due to secondary changes that accompany pregnancy disruption (necrosis of decidual and tropho-blastic tissue and inflammation which act to stimulate the generation of endogenous PG, see also Chapter Three).

The emergence of an alternative explanation of RU 486 action does not modify our rejection of it as an abortifacient. Rather, it justifies our opinion that antiprogesterones are poorly understood and their application as abortifacients is ill-conceived. Schering, the German pharmaceutical company responsible for developing the ZK analogues, has refrained from entering the commercial market, perhaps due to threats from the anti-abortion lobby. However, it is equally likely that the theoretical uncertainty surrounding the basic concept of antiprogesterone-induced abortion accounts for the company's unwillingness to proceed, particularly since the Roussel Uclaf proposed mechanism of action was challenged by experimental data obtained from the research laboratories of Schering in Berlin. Schering has advised us that the company has no present intention to market chemicals for abortion purpose, at least not in the United States, Canada or Mexico. However research and development of the Schering antiprogestin substance is continuing for the 'treatment of illnesses such as breast cancer and endometriosis' (pers. comm. to LD and RK).[6] This, of course, does not rule out the future re-entry of the ZK analogues into the abortifacient market.

Epostane, another antiprogesterone, was originally developed for abortion purposes, but at present its commercial marketing has been suspended. It is a synthetic steroid which acts to block the enzyme 3ß-hydroxysteroid dehydrogenase and thereby inhibit progesterone synthesis to induce abortion. The physiological and clinical effects of epostane have been determined in first-trimester pregnancy termination procedures carried out in Australia, the Netherlands, Sweden and the UK.

Results from the Netherlands experience of epostane (Crooij *et al.*, 1988) were featured in the Digest section of *Perspectives in Family Planning* (September/October, 1988: 241) under a headline which is now exceedingly familiar, 'New treatment to end early pregnancy found to be safe and effective'. Here the effective complete abortion rate was somewhat higher, 84 per cent, than that achieved in other epostane studies. Yet, in what was lauded to be safe and effective, two women (4%), of the mere 50 treated, suffered serious complications that necessitated a blood transfusion for one, and dilatation and curettage on day 20 for the other. A further eight women (16%) did not respond to treatment, (referred to as 'non-responders'), and subsequently underwent dilatation and curettage 'without complication'. From a woman's perspective these ineffective attempts to induce abortion are in themselves serious complications. As such, failed treatments increase the frequency of serious complications to 20 per cent rather than the reported four per cent. Further, if the 76 per cent of women who are reported to find epostane preferable to dilatation and curettage are viewed from a critical direction, this represents non-approval from one woman in every four. It does not require too much imagination to predict that the 20 per cent of women, judged by our criteria to have experienced severe complication(s), are significantly represented within the reported 24 per cent of women who did not prefer epostane to a conventional abortion.

A comparison of the consequences of epostane administered during a first trimester pregnancy termination with those from RU 486 was reported from a study of Swedish women by Odlind and Birgerson (1987). The complete abortion rate was 73 per cent in the epostane-treated women, compared with only 61 per cent in two RU 486 treatment groups. Adverse effects were, however, more frequent in the epostane-treated women, with nausea and/or vomiting, together with pain and headache, resulting from RU 486 and epostane. In terms of complete abortion, these results were reported to 'clearly indicate' that neither epostane nor the RU 486 method was superior to vacuum aspiration or PG treatment. This comment supports our major contention that RU 486 is not an improved abortion method when compared with PG-induced terminations. And since conventional abortion methods are markedly preferable to those using PGs, support for a chemical cocktail which includes both RU 486 and a PG analogue, is an illogical and unreasonable expectation.

While epostane has been shelved and the ZK analogues placed in reserve, RU 486 has survived and continues to be promoted, due in no mean part to the extraordinary efforts of its prime-mover, Etienne Baulieu, rather than its scientific merit. As such its days are limited to the point where the rhetoric ceases to shelter a pill that was mistakenly identified as 'a miracle'. In fact, new RU 486/PG 'cocktails' continue

to emerge, one 'perfectly timed' to counter the announce-
ment of a young French woman's death following the
administration of RU 486 plus *'a small dose of sulprostone'* in
April 1991. Baulieu informed the French Academy of
Sciences that he had devised a simpler way to use the RU
486 abortion pill, with the 'off-label' application of the oral
PG analogue, misoprostol. He revealed that he has already
obtained results in 100 women which confirm the safety of
'RU 486 plus a small dose of misoprostol' (Altman, 1991). Yet
misoprostol's manufacturer, G. D. Searle (USA), on the
insert that is placed into each package in its North American
distribution, warns: 'Cytotec (misoprostol) must not be
used by pregnant women. Cytotec may cause miscarriages.
Miscarriages caused by Cytotec may be incomplete and
could lead to dangerous bleeding'. Indeed, Baulieu's results
from 100 women were reported to include five abortion
failures (5%). The embryo was incompletely expelled in
four women whose abortions were completed by
conventional method over the next 10 days. The fifth
pregnancy continued.

A Searle representative informed us that they, like the
Schering Company, had no intention to market misoprostol
for abortion purposes (pers. comm. to LD, 17 April 1991).
This means that women are not guaranteed any greater
safety from misoprostol than they were from the 'off-label'
use of sulprostone with RU 486. Further, Searle informed
us that misoprostol has only minimal uterine effects, which
are in fact inferior to those of another oral Searle PG
analogue, enisoprost.

We have been concerned for some time that misoprostol
was being used in a South American country to terminate
unwanted pregnancies. Specifically, in countries where
abortion is illegal, information is not compiled to identify
the hazards from the 'off-label' use of certain drugs as
abortifacients (Dumble, 1991). It was recently reported
that there was growing abuse of misoprostol as an
abortifacient in Brazil (Schönhöfer, 1991). At the maternity

hospital in Fortazela, Brazil, misoprostol was named as the inducing agent in 73 per cent of 525 pregnant women seeking emergency treatment for uterine bleeding in 1990 (p. 1535). Abortion was incomplete 'about half of the time', thereby exposing women and their fetuses to untold health perils. Within the preliminary report of misoprostol abortion failures, and additional to the emergency medical requirements of the women, five babies were born with large skin and bone defects on the frontal part of the skull that left the brain exposed. Surgical closure of the open defect was attempted within four days of birth but all infants experienced convulsions and infections (one fatal). These are merely the short-term complications, but as Schönhöfer, too, concluded, any society that prohibits legal abortion will encounter illicit drug usage to induce uterine expulsion. We would argue that RU 486 *plus a small dose of misoprostol* is no more immune to 'illegal' use than misoprostol has been as a single drug.

Perhaps Etienne Baulieu did not choose enisoprost for his most recent experiment because of its higher incidence of gastrointestinal side-effects. Alternatively, he could have chosen to extend the data of Swahn *et al.*, 1990, who, almost a year earlier, had *published* abortion details of RU 486 with the oral PG analogue, 9-methylene PGE_2. The latter would certainly have been a more conscionable approach than his promotion of misoprostol as an abortifacient, an application for which it is neither intended nor successful. Instead, in his self-ordained 'work to give women more choices' (Delaney, 1991), he has opted to establish yet another health hazard for women from the unknown effect(s) of a further untested chemical cocktail. At this stage we can only ask how many more health hazards will be contrived before RU 486/PG-based abortion is finally abandoned – at worst a misconception, at best, a myth?

Conclusion

There is much about RU 486/PG that is fraught with risk and problems. As we have queried, what is the meaning of a 'private' and 'de-medicalized' abortion that requires three or four doctor's visits to a specialized centre, includes the taking of two and perhaps five hazardous drug combinations, is accompanied by vaginal ultrasound, and too often has complications ranging from moderate bleeding to severe pain and, for some women, blood transfusions? If this is a private and de-medicalized abortion experience, then the word 'private' has lost its definitional moorings.

There is a sense of unreality about this doublespeak that on the one hand, promotes RU 486/PG as a simple pill that can be popped in the privacy of a woman's home and, on the other hand, states quite clearly that it will never be given without strict medical supervision. There is also an intentional doublespeak that governs the representation of how RU 486 acts to affect reproduction.

The promoters of RU 486 are deliberately blurring the line between contraception and abortion. When tested as a contraceptive, RU 486 is problematic because it interferes with the next menstrual cycle and leads to disturbances of monthly cycles (Nieman and Loriaux, 1988). It has also been acknowledged that 'the drug is not suitable as a routine postcoital birth-control agent' (Ulmann *et al.*, 1990: 48). Instead, Baulieu uses the term 'contragestive' to avoid, as he states, the negative and guilt-producing associations of the word abortion. He insists that his research 'is not aimed at gaining women abortions,' but 'at helping them control gestation' (quoted in Gardner, 1989: 6). This is comparable to the reproductive technologists performing the linguistic feat of turning a less-than-fourteen day embryo into a 'pre-embryo' so as to justify embryo experimentation.

Doublespeak is an attempt to make the negative appear positive, as in the claim that RU 486 medicalization is de-medicalization, and strict medical supervision is privacy. Doublespeak also makes the complications appear minimal, or at least tolerable. Finally, doublespeak is a language that curbs thinking and acute questioning, as evidenced in the lack of any critical perspective offered by many women's groups.

There are many reasons why individual women and women's groups have jumped on the RU 486/PG band-wagon. The packaging of the new abortifacient has been immensely successful. 'The very nature of the specialized knowledge and information, the complexity of the technology, the way the 'advances' have been publicized in the popular media and such places as *Science* magazine, and the incredibly slick marketing job which is being done, have had the effect of silencing criticism' (pers. comm. to JR from Judy Luce, June 1991).

Many women's groups have taken the erosion of women's right to abortion, as well as the fear of playing into the hands of the right-wing, as incentive enough for promoting RU 486/PG. The philosophy prevails that 'we' – those who are committed to women's rights – must be *for* whatever 'they' – those who are not committed to women's rights, i.e. the anti-abortionists – are against. However, this defense of RU 486/PG has been too much defined by a reaction to the right wing.

It has been the purpose of this report to demonstrate that many of the basic assumptions about RU 486/PG abortion need to be fundamentally re-examined. In light of the misleading claims and the various complications, we ask if these drugs are an appropriate abortion technology for women. Environmental engineer, Pat Hynes has elsewhere raised the crucial question that 'As a wave of green logos and lifestyle washes over industrial countries, making people conscious of not putting any unnecessary synthetic chemical substances on and into their body, why are women being advised to use synthetic' drugs (Hynes, 1990: 20)? The issue here is not that these drugs are synthetic, but that most of these reproductive drugs used to intervene in women's reproductive cycle often have serious risks and complications. Thus for the last quarter of a century, feminist health activists have been put in the position of risk management and risk communication, documenting the downside of such technologies and drugs. At the same time, reproductive technologists, while admitting that there are some risks, minimize them so that the technologies and drugs become acceptable and go forward, despite the complications. They offer studies that convince women that the risks can be managed and that if women want effective contraception, abortions, and children, the risks have to be lived with.

At a time when the rest of the planet is being warned about the risks of chemical fixes, there is an enormous increase in the number and kinds of drugs that are being prescribed for women, especially in the reproductive realm. From a girl's birth to a woman's death, she is often prescribed fertility drugs, the pill, a new generation of anti-pregnancy vaccines that are especially being promoted in third world countries, tranquilizers, estrogen – currently, hormone – replacement therapy, and now RU 486/PG, a haphazard combination of two dubious drugs. Given the short period during which RU 486/PG is effective (albeit poorly), 10–40 per cent of the fertilized eggs/early embryos might be expelled through spontaneous abortion and would *not* require any chemical intervention. Thus, RU 486/PG may be unwarranted in a significant number of women. Calculated at the 30 per cent level, this could amount to 18,000 of the 60,000 French women so treated! Can we be disturbed about chemically fed plants and animals and remain unconcerned about chemically fed women?

There *is* a dearth of research, development, and implementation of birth control, abortion, and reproductive technology as the promoters of RU 486 claim. What is more important, however, is that there is a dearth of *appropriate technology* for women. And most of the technology that has been developed requires medical supervision and control. There has been a virtual non-existence of research into condom improvement, barrier methods, and menstrual extraction, in contrast to the enthusiasm for the pill, IUDs, injectables, and sterilization. Most of the reproductive technology and drugs thus far, as well as those now being proposed, are attended by risk, harm and, in some cases, death to women.

People expect and accept technological solutions as unmitigated progress. The history of the medicalization of reproduction in the west has spawned the biomedical control of women's reproductive lives, the technological and surgical management of pregnancy and childbirth, and the development and continued use of questionable drugs and technologies. RU 486/PG cannot be seen apart from this history of technological fixes and medical control of women's lives.

For example, why are the abortion options in most western countries completely medicalized? We see this again with RU 486, although the rhetoric of demedicalization is emphasized. Without exception, however, every physician now working with the drug emphasizes that strict medical supervision is necessary. Strict medical supervision is also strict medical control. When the American Medical Association voted to support the testing of the drug in the United States, it stated: 'This is not an abortion issue; this is an issue of scientific research for a drug that can be useful for many different medical problems' (Lee, 1990: 2). The Association feared that women's health activists would import the drug, and delegates supporting the resolution lamented that the drug would be used without proper medical supervision. The other side of this fear is that RU 486/PG would be launched outside the parameters of medical control.

The push for medical control of abortion is in keeping with the historical position of doctors in the west toward all forms of reproductive technologies, including birthing and birth control, as well as abortion methods. Historically, it was the medical lobby that influenced law and public policy, keeping birth control and abortion under the control of physicians. Robert Dickinson, a leading advocate for gynecologists in the early 20th century, who promoted contraception with Margaret Sanger, urged his physician colleagues to keep birth control in their own hands and not let it go to the radicals (Gordon, 1976: 249–300). The radicals, of course, were mostly women who were demanding birth control along with political and legal change. Many of these women succumbed to the pressure promoting physician control and the strict medicalization of birth control. Ultimately, when birth control was approved in the United States, legislation mandated that only *doctors* could import, mail, and dispense it.

Reproductive technological history seems to be repeating itself. The current feminist campaigns for abortion and for RU 486/PG seem confined in this same straitjacket of advocating for abortion choices for women, but within the boundaries established by the medical profession and population planners. Population organizations, such as the Population Crisis Committee and the Population Council, the developer of Norplant, have sponsored research on RU 486/PG and are promoting its distribution.

Of concern is the current promotional collaboration

between population control groups, pharmaceutical and medical researchers, and women's groups – all of whom have coalesced to support the development and distribution of the abortifacient, especially in the United States. This recent co-operation between population policy and planning groups and feminists sparked a heated and acrimonious debate at the 6th International Women and Health Meeting, held in the Philippines in November 1990. Many women, particularly those from developing countries, question this collaboration as not in women's health and political interests. 'I fear that we are just going to share in a power which uses our speeches, but does not change the practices and the reality which that power imposes, and which, coincidentally, are what we started out fighting against, from the standpoint of reproductive rights' (de la Fuente, 1989: 3).

One of the historical legacies of the women's health movement of the 60s and 70s was the de-medicalization of a wide range of health practices. The emphasis was put on techniques/technology which reduced the need for medical supervision. Self-help was not merely a slogan but was translated into examining one's own cervix, developing menstrual extraction methods, and treating yeast infections, to name but a few of the procedures. Obviously, self-help was not enough when confronted with the fact that many women have no access to self-help education and depend upon institutionalized medicine. But the feminist critique knew the difference between a procedure which gave women real control of their bodies and a chemical cocktail attended by all the accoutrements of extensive medical-technical intervention.

Abortion is one of the simplest of presently medicalized gynecological procedures, requiring less expertise, training, and skill than attending births. Trained paramedics in third world countries perform abortions safely and competently. Why then cannot trained lay women do abortions in western non-medical contexts? Rather than advocating for one more dubious reproductive technology such as RU 486/PG, feminists should be fighting for de-medicalizing conventional abortion methods, and doctors and family planning groups should be joining suit.

The only US states where abortion can be legally performed by non-physicians are Vermont and Montana. Yet doctors in the United States are not required to learn to perform abortions. Only one in four of physicians-in-training learn the technique. In rural areas, the number of doctors and clinics performing abortions has been halved since 1977 (The Guttmacher Institute quoted in Goodman, 1990: 91). In the US anti-abortion climate, many doctors have ceased to perform abortions, and others will never perform them. Many people, even physicians, believe that the answer to the abortion problem is to train non-physicians to do abortions (US ABC News, 1990). This does not mean that physicians should not perform abortions, or that the medical foundation for abortion services is dispensable. It *does* mean that abortions need not only, or chiefly, be done by doctors.

The Vermont Women's Health Centre performs one-third of all abortions in that state. All are done by physicians' assistants who, as part of a two-year training program in women's health care, learn the procedure. Their record of safety and frequency of complications is slightly better than physician-performed abortions (US ABC News, 1990). In many countries throughout the world, trained lay practitioners are increasingly involved in modern abortion treatment. Midwives and other lay practitioners perform early abortions. We can learn much from lay midwives in making the case for women-controlled abortions. For it is lay midwives, more than others, who have led the way in de-medicalizing reproduction.

Pauline Bart's article on the Jane Collective, 'Seizing the Means of Reproduction: a Feminist Abortion Collective: How and Why It Worked,' is virtually the only published work available on lay abortion practitioners in the United

States. This article, appearing in *Qualitative Sociology* (1987: 339–56), documented and described the work of Jane in Chicago. Jane functioned as an illegal abortion service working out of private apartments from 1969–1973, until some of its founders decided that the 1973 US Supreme Court decision made the service obsolete. Others connected with Jane felt that the service never should have stopped doing abortions, because nobody did them better. Even in the few months after the US Supreme Court legalized abortions, Jane was receiving over 300 calls a week (Elze, 1988: 12). Over the course of four years, they performed 11,000 abortions at various stages of pregnancy. Their safety record for first trimester abortions was equal to that of New York State after 1973, following the legalization of abortion there (Clement, 1983: 10).

During the 1970s, many women's self-help groups practiced a technique know as menstrual extraction. Initially developed by Lorraine Rothman and women at the Los Angeles Self Help Clinic in 1971, menstrual extraction gently removes by suction the contents of the uterus on or about the first day of menstruation. Using a flexible plastic cannula attached to a bottle, an automatic valve attachment controls the direction of the air flow and locks in the pressure, eliminating any possibility of pushing menstrual fluid or air back into the uterus (Rothman, 1978: 45). No uterine perforations, infection, or air embolisms resulted, as have occurred at times with physicians who use dilators, large rigid cannulas and curettes (*ibid.*, 48). Obviously, this technique depends upon women engaging in self-help groups and being part of an ongoing contingent of women dedicated to learning and practising the technique with each other. However, there is no reason why more women cannot learn menstrual extraction and begin to practice it in self-help groups as happened earlier.

Abortion is not a complicated procedure. If women could learn to be midwives attending birth and performing a wider range of complex and skilled procedures, even more women could learn to do abortions. As the Jane Collective demonstrated, it is possible to provide safe, skilled, caring and inexpensive abortions by trained lay women in non-medical settings, outside the medical monopoly.

This report has been critical of RU 486/PG abortion. At the same time, however, we believe that it is important to speak about alternatives, especially in a context where conventional abortion options are increasingly under siege by anti-abortion fundamentalists. It is our contention that feminists must challenge the hegemonic physician provision of abortions, a monopoly that lacks credibility as decreasing numbers of doctors are trained/skilled to perform abortions. Rather than doctors enlisting feminists to fight for one more debilitating and dangerous technology, why aren't feminists recruiting physicians, family planners, and others to de-medicalize abortion when it seems to be in the best interests of women and doctors who, in large measure, do not want to do abortions to begin with?

More is at stake, in abortion, than a technological choice. Jacqueline Darroch Forrest, the chief of research for the Alan Guttmacher Institute, says, 'We are fooling ourselves if we think a technological fix is going to get us out of our dilemma of high rates of pregnancy and abortion' (quoted in Hilts, 1990: 55). In our view, this dilemma raises more political and philosophical issues that feminists must address concerning women's sexual and reproductive self-determination. RU 486/PG represents the epitome of a reproductive politics that makes no connection to the sexual politics of women's lives. Women alone bear the burden of these drugs and technology. All of the medicalized methods have absolved men of reproductive responsibility. In fact, RU 486 may absolve men of any future contraceptive commitment since the drug has been promoted as 'safe and easy' for women. Thus many men may view its availability as more comfortable (for them) than using condoms. There is no recognition of what Catharine MacKinnon has called 'a whole net of relations in which [women] are (at present) inescapably gendered...' and in which '...the struggle for reproductive freedom has never included a woman's right to refuse sex...' (MacKinnon, 1987: 98).

Instead the focus has been on RU 486/PG as a woman's choice and as part of her right to privacy. The emphasis here is on access for women to any kind of abortion, unaccompanied by any analysis of women's access to an independent sexuality freed from male definition, male access to women's bodies, and risk to women's health and well-being. 'I wonder if a woman can be presumed to control access to her sexuality if she feels unable to interrupt intercourse to insert a diaphragm; or worse, cannot even want to, aware that she risks a pregnancy she knows she does not want...Abortion policy has never been explicitly approached in the context of how women get pregnant...' (MacKinnon, 1987: 96).

Feminists cannot advocate for reproductive freedom without advocating that women control their sexuality. Critics of abortion restrictions, for example, cannot ignore why women need abortions to begin with: because they cannot refuse sex; because they have sex forced on them; because they are raped; because they are prostituted; because they are young girls made pregnant by fathers, brothers or male relatives who use them sexually; because they are teenagers who have sex but don't know why; because they are women who accidentally or unintentionally become pregnant; because contraception fails, because they lack not only basic sex education but basic sexual freedom; and because of all the other conditions present in a context of women's oppression.

The issues surrounding RU 486/PG are not only part of the 'politics of reproduction' but of 'sexual politics' as well. As with other issues of sexual politics, here, too, we must address access to women and the abuse of women's bodies

– for medical research and experimentation, for clinical experience, and for financial gain under the heading of scientific advancement and treatment 'for our own good.'

Choice has become the reigning value on the pro-abortion front. Pro-choice, not pro-woman, has become the slogan for groups acting to protect abortion rights for women in western countries. It is almost as if the rhetoric of choice might attract those who are not sure about their commitment to women's rights but are definitely committed to the right to choose. Choice resonates as a quintessential US value. This report contends that feminist reliance on a rhetoric of choice lacks not only honesty, but vision and aspiration. It also allows for all sorts of things to be defended in the name of choice – prostitution, pornography, surrogate contracts, and the gamut of reproductive technologies – without any genuine recognition of how such choices deprive many women of autonomy, dignity, integrity, well-being, and basic social justice. The emphasis on choice narrows the questions surrounding abortion, so that how abortion fits into the total oppression of women is rarely discussed.

No procedure requiring strict medical supervision and involving a host of risks and complications will help provide sexual and reproductive self-determination for women. On the macro level, women must make the connections between sexual and reproductive freedom. On the micro level, rather than depending on some medical miracle to guarantee abortion rights for women, this report advocates that women should 'seize the means of reproduction' and act in our best interests.

ENDNOTES

Chapter One

1   The patent license for RU 486 does not include Baulieu. This is interesting since Baulieu is hailed, worldwide, as the 'father' of RU 486.

2   Judith Vincent from *Sojourner* comments on this question in 1990:

> There is also the possibility that a combination pill could be manufactured, but the patent for such a pill is held by Schering, a German pharmaceutical company. Schering has approached Roussel about working together, but Roussel isn't interested. To complicate matters, Schering has developed a drug similar to RU 486 – too similar. Roussel claims infringement on its patent rights (Vincent, 1990: 11H). (For further comments on these other drugs see Chapter Four).

3   Exceptions are Maria *et al.*, (1988); Sitruk-Ware *et al.*, (1990); Somell and Ölund (1990).

4   Interestingly, the two preferred prostaglandins – sulprostone (Nalador) and gemeprost (Cervagem) – are manufactured by Schering AG, Berlin and May and Baker, Degenham, UK, thus undercutting Roussel Uclaf's position as solo drug provider for chemical abortion.

5   A previous paper published in 1988 from the same study had only mentioned 160 women (Gao *et al.*).

6   In 1990, an unpublished Roussel Uclaf paper lists 10,250 women (Aubeny, 1990).

7   According to Allan Templeton who prepared the 1990 UK Multitrial report, the results are 'an interim analysis for a larger study of more than 1000 patients'.

8   It is also alleged that Wolfgang Hilger, President of Hoechst, the German pharmaceutical company which owns 54.5 per

cent of Roussel Uclaf, opposed the marketing of the pill for anti-abortionist reasons (Kingman, 1989).

9   Roussel scientist, André Ulmann, was quoted in *The Washington Post* on 3 October as saying that despite the fact that the drug had received government approval earlier in 1988, his company would not be marketing the product in China 'at least for the time being' unless the Chinese government made an official request (Herman, 1988: 12). Originally Roussel Uclaf also ceased to pursue marketing approval in Great Britain, Sweden and Holland. Earlier in 1988, it had withdrawn RU 486 from an Australian research project to test the drug on 40 pregnant women at Monash Medical Centre under the direction of David Healy, a supporter of RU 486 and PG, as part of the WHO multicenter trials. (David Healy hopes to have the drug returned by September/October 1991.) In fact, the Australian Federal Health Department had been deliberating for seven months, when Roussel Uclaf withdrew the application (Hills, 1988: 3). In 1989, Roussel Uclaf also withdrew its drug from the Los Angeles County Hospital where David Grimes and others had conducted the only US trials, and experiments ceased in February 1990.

10   With the exception of some critical statements by feminists, objections to RU 486 are coming mainly from people who are opposed to chemical abortion on anti-abortion grounds and do not engage with its many dangers for women. An exception was a working paper based on medical articles which, in addition to its anti-abortion stance, listed some of the actual and potential adverse effects on women by Nick Tonti-Filippini, former Director of St Vincent's Bioethics Centre, Melbourne, now Research Officer for the Australian Catholic Bishops' Conference (Tonti-Filippini, 1990).

11   Interviews with Lynette Dumble, Renate Klein and Jocelynne Scutt by Kerry O'Brien, 'Lateline TV', (ABC, 15.11.90); Anne Delaney, 'The Health Report', (ABC Sydney, 19.11.90 and 22.4.91); Ruth Barney, 'Women on the Line' (3CR Melbourne, 25.11.90 and 18.5.91); Cecily McNeill 'Good Morning NZ', (Radio New Zealand, 20.11.90); Matthew

Abraham (ABC Canberra, 8.5.91); Jackie Fitzgerald (ABC Perth, 9.5.91).

12   The *Journal Officiel* published the decision concerning the fixed price for chemical abortion on 25 February 1990. Eighty per cent of the costs are rebatable from the French National Health Service. It does not mention whether, should an additional conventional pregnancy termination be necessary, this is included in the total abortion cost.

13   An article in the *New Scientist* in May 1990 dismissed the intervention by the international committee calling it an anti-abortionist group (Hughes, 1990: 3). We have not been able to verify their claim. None of the French articles on this group made any reference to their supposed anti-abortion stance. In fact the group's statement does not dismiss conventional abortion but rather condemns chemical abortion as an inferior alternative.

14   Speaking at a meeting in New Zealand, Etienne Baulieu reported a very low incidence of complications. An Auckland gynecologist remarked that these figures were inconsistent with his own extensive reading of the literature. As journalist Sandra Coney pointed out, what had happened was that Baulieu quoted side-effects reported by women at follow-up visits eight to twelve days *after* the RU 486 was given rather than at the time of administration! (Coney, 1990a: 11).

15   This part of Nissim's letter was omitted by Marge Berer.

16   Other critical articles appeared in the Australian Healthsharing Women *Newsletter* (Moore, 1990), *Inkwell Newsletter* of the Women's Electoral Lobby (Klein, 1991), *The Age* (Cafarella, 1991), *Broadsheet*, New Zealand (Fidler, 1991), *Emanzipation*, Switzerland (1991), *Spare Rib*, UK (Raymond, 1991) and *Vogue USA* (Ince, 1991).

17   Baulieu, furthermore, called LD 'ill-read' on 'Nightline TV' and delivered a diatribe against an interview with RK, calling her facts 'untrue' and her critical questions 'a waste of time' and doubting her credentials to speak on the issue of RU 486: 'Maybe she is a dentist who likes to speak about the bad gastric surgery . . . Should I give a talk because I am a doctor

about neurosurgery when I am a hormone specialist? I think this way not to know a matter and to speak of it covered by the title "Doctor" is just irresponsible' (Transcript Newztel: 2). Asked by the interviewer why he was so defensive about legitimate questions relating to a new drug, his response was that he was not defensive but offensive [*sic*!] but he did not 'like somebody who hides some untold prejudice behind . . . let's say the heart of a doctor' (p. 10). These comments prompted the interviewer to hastily bring the broadcast to an end commenting, 'well we may be at risk of defamation here, Professor Baulieu, so those are your words and certainly not Radio New Zealand's' (p. 10). In a later interview with Anne Delaney on the Health Report, Radio National in Australia (22.4.91) he described her questions as slightly vicious and discontinued the telephone conversation, because, as he put it, he had to continue his work for women!

18 Baulieu is *not* the first to use an oral prostaglandin. Swahn *et al.* published a study with an oral prostaglandin in 1990.

Chapter Three

1 This is one of the many places in medical literature where the inherent sexism of this profession expresses itself overtly by conceptualizing a woman's body as a militaristic site – a 'target' – and an incubator for a pregnancy – hence in this case the 'rescue' of the doomed 'curious' corpus luteum by a fertilized egg!

2 From our perspective, Arpad Istvan Csapo is central to the conceptualization of chemical abortion. His concepts and recommendations provided the background for contemporary chemical abortion and the threat it poses to women. He was born in Hungary in 1918, where he received his medical degree (an MD) and initial medical appointment at the University of Szeged. He was an Associate Professor at the Rockefeller Institute from 1956–1961 and chief of its laboratory of reproductive physiology from 1961–1963. In 1961 he was appointed as Professor of Obstetrics and Gynecology at Washington University, St Louis, Missouri. He was also the

Mannheimer Fellow at the University of Uppsala, Sweden, 1948–49; Fellow of the Carnegie Institute, USA, 1949–51; Fellow of the Guggenheim Institute, USA, 1954–55; Lecturer in Gynecology and Obstetrics at John Hopkins University, 1951; the CIBA Lecturer at the University of London, UK, 1952; and an Honorary Professor at Bahia University, Brazil, 1958. He was awarded the De Snoovan't Foundation Prize in 1964 for research in reproductive physiology (*American Men and Women in Science*, 1976).

3 The question is never asked what actually happens to *RU 486* once it has taken the place of progesterone.

4 Initially the half-life of RU 486 was believed to be only around 10 hours (Bertagna *et al.*, 1984: 27).

5 Earlier, in a 1988 publication, Baulieu simply stated that 'In a woman's body, the half-life of RU 486 is approx. 20 h' – thus making the reader believe that this figure was based on conclusive research (p. 125).

6 One of the few RU 486 studies which investigate its effect on the hypothalamus is a report from Sheffield, UK (Li *et al.*,1988) which reports 23 per cent mood changes, irritability, depression and marked thirst sensation in women who had received RU 486 in the luteal phase for menstrual induction.

7 See Schreiber *et al.* (1983); Deraedt *et al.* (1985) and Heikinheimo *et al.* (1986) for studies on the pharmakinetics of RU 486 in rats, men and women. Many of their results are contradictory and inconclusive, and the papers end with the demand for further research. Furthermore, similar studies investigating the *mutual* actions of RU 486 and prostaglandins upon one another have not been undertaken.

8 Progestagen-only pills also cause menstrual disturbances, a reduction of tubal motility, 'persistent and/or heavy bleeding', amenorrhea due to anovulation, mastalgia (sore breasts) and headaches that are said to be 'not uncommon' (Kleinman, 1990: 64).

9 In his article about the prevention of cardiovascular risk in women Michael Kafrissen specifically mentions the proges-

tin levonorgestrel as severely implicated in cardiovascular risk for women because of its strong androgenicity (1990: 18). Levonorgestrel is the synthetic hormone in Norplant. It is scandalous that this serious shortcoming did not prevent the US FDA from approving Norplant in December 1990 and was not mentioned in the positive publicity for the drug.

10 The anterior pituitary also produces prolactin (which stimulates the breast to produce milk). According to Swahn *et al.* (1989) and the WHO Taskforce multicenter trial (1989), after RU 486 administration prolactin levels rose and did not decrease after the abortion (p. 724): a further unexplained and concerning effect of this drug.

11 Since RU 486 has been described as an agonist of progesterone, research might reveal that it also acts as an agonist of androgen. If this were the case, RU 486 treatment could lead to an increase in testosterone in women.

12 In 1989, Etienne-Emile Baulieu was awarded the Lasker Award rumored by some to be the precursor of the Nobel prize.

13 Glaucoma, i.e. intraocular pressure, has been lowered in rabbits after the administration of RU 486 (Phillips *et al.*, 1984).

14 It is worth quoting Stuenkel *et al.*'s research design (1990) in full as it is a particularly crude example of medical science's ruthlessness in using women's bodies as test-sites. It is but one example but testifies to the invasiveness of ill-conceived and poorly designed research. Stuenkel *et al.* recruited five 'normally cycling women' with 'ideal' body weights who had not used hormonal contraception for at least 6 months. They write:

> Studies were conducted during three consecutive menstrual cycles consisting of a control cycle, treatment cycle and recovery cycle. Beginning on the first day of menses (day 1), *daily blood samples* were drawn throughout the study for measurements of LH, follicle stimulating hormone (FSH), estradiol (E2) and P. On day 3 of the control cycle, LH pulsatility was assessed in four of five

women by *10 minute frequent blood sampling for 10 hours.* During the treatment cycle, RU 486 was administered at a dose of 3 mg/kg orally, once a day for three days, beginning on the 1st or 2nd day of menses. On the third day of RU 486 administration, *10 minute frequent blood sampling for 10 hours was repeated* in the same four women. Each frequent blood sampling study was performed *after an overnight fast.* One hour after insertion of an indwelling *intravenous catheter,* blood sampling was begun. Mealtimes were approximately 8:00 A.M., 12.00 noon, and 5.00 P.M. *Subjects were not allowed to smoke or sleep during the frequent sampling'* (p. 643, our emphasis).

15 RU 486 has been found to inhibit fertilization in mice. Juneja and Dodson (1990) unsuccessfully tried to reverse the decreased hCG production by adding progesterone (as suggested by Das and Catt (1987) and conclude that, 'The inhibition of fertilization is mediated through a progesterone independent mechanism or the binding of progesterone is non-reversible' (p. 220); see also Yang and Wu, this chapter.

16 It is interesting to note that a number of prominent infertility specialists/IVF doctors also promote RU 486/PG and are involved in its research. Among them are: Gary Hodgen, USA; René Frydman, France; Allan Templeton, UK; David Healy, Australia. Their uncritical attitudes towards the adverse effects from fertility drugs are revisited in their praise for this latest technological 'fix'.

17 To their surprise they also found that follicles developed during the administration of the antiprogestin NET: a result that raises questions about the role of progesterone in follicle development. In addition they noted that no decline in the FSH and LH concentrations took place; a finding which contrasted with those of Shoupe *et al.,* 1987; Nieman *et al.,* 1986 and Di Mattina, 1987.

18 The manufacturers of clomiphene citrate, Merrill Dow (Clomid) and Serono (Serophene), state clearly that 50 mg per day is the preferred dose which could be extended to 100mg, and occasionally to 150 mg but for three days only.

Administration for five days is thus clearly unacceptable. But even more outrageous is the fact that clomiphene, which has many proven short- and long-term adverse effects, is administered to perfectly healthy ovulating women!

19 The main finding from this study was 'that progesterone is not critical for the final stages of oocyte maturation' (p. 592).

20 Furthermore, they observed perivitelline *polyspermy* in both unfertilized and fertilized eggs (e.g. an accumulation of sperm between the zona pellucida and the vitelline membrane of the inner part of the egg). In fertilized eggs perivitelline polyspermy 'increased from 10.7 per cent (control) to 54.9 per cent, 73.6 per cent and 83.3 per cent' at three different RU 486 concentrations (p. 218).

21 Yang and Wu list four other studies on rats and mice which also showed adverse effects from RU486 on embryo development. In all of them, however, RU 486 was administered by injection whilst their own study used oral administration as is the case in women.

22 The cited third case of a woman who received RU 486 but vomited one and a half hours later (and reported seeing pills) is totally inappropriate to prove 'normal' development after *exposure* to RU 486!

Chapter Four

1 Eicosanoid molecules result from the metabolism of arachidonic acid, with several distinct forms of prostaglandin (also spoken of as prostanoids) being produced from the cyclooxygenase metabolic pathway, and leukotrienes from the lipoxygenase pathway. The chemical abbreviations for the prostaglandins discussed in this report are as follows: PGE_1 (prostaglandin E_1), PGE_2 (prostaglandin E_2), $PGF_{2\alpha}$ (prostaglandin $F_{2\alpha}$) and PGI_2 (prostacyclin).

2 'Off-label' prescription of drugs, following their licensing for a specified purpose (which is 'on-label' prescription), is entirely at the discretion of the physician and falls outside

the authority of the government bureau and pharmaceutical company responsible for the drug licence application.

3 The diverse, and often totally opposite, functions of prostaglandins are not unique to their interactions with ovarian hormones. Another such example is the outcome of prostaglandin interactions with lymphocytes (the white blood cells responsible for immune protection) where dosage manipulations permit the induction of either immunosuppression or immunostimulation. Taken together with the variation in individual sensitivity to prostaglandins, the contradictory effects of both exogenous and endogenous prostaglandins are further evidence that RU 486/PG abortion methods should be resisted.

4 The type of prostaglandin analogue, its dose, administration site and infusion time, and the number of previous pregnancies, are each factors which contribute to the abortion-rate in prostaglandin-induced terminations.

5 The guinea pig model was also crucial to the discovery of sulprostone, which had very little activity in the rat model. Its therapeutic potential would not have been recognized, but for guinea-pig studies which identified 'E-prostaglandins to be more potent abortifacients than F-prostaglandins' (Elger *et al.*, 1987: 79). Subsequent studies in the guinea-pig model indicated the following ascending order of abortifacient activity: $PGF_{2\alpha}$, PGE_2, PGE_1, sulprostone/15-methyl-$PGF_{2\alpha}$ and 16,16-dimethyl-PGE_2 which paralleled to a considerable extent the order of effectiveness observed in human pregnancy.

6 K. Schmidt-Gollwitzer from Schering Gynecological Therapy replied to our questions of 22 January 1991 with the following statement: 'We are conducting research on and developing anti-progestin substances for the treatment of illnesses such as breast cancer or endometriosis. The substances presently under development are not intended for the indication of abortion' (pers. comm. to LD and RK, 19 March 1991).

BIBLIOGRAPHY

ABC Nightly News Special Report with Peter Jennings. (1990). 29 November, USA.

Altman, Lawrence K. (1991, 9 April). A simpler way to employ RU 498 is reported. *New York Times*. C3

American Men and Women in Science. (1976). Thirteenth edition. R.R. Bawker Company: New York.

Asch, Ricardo H., Weckstein, Louis N., Balmaceda, Jose P., Rojas, Francisco, Spitz, Irving M. and Tadir, Yona. (1990). Case Report. Non-surgical expulsion of non-viable pregnancy: a new application of RU 486. *Human Reproduction 5* (4): 481–483.

Atrash, Hani, Lawson, Herschel W. and Smith, Jack C. (1990). Legal Abortion in the US: Trends and Mortality. *Contemporary OB/GYN* (February): 58–69.

Aubeny, Elisabeth. (1990). New Perspectives for Patients: Drug Induced Abortion by RU 486 and Prostaglandins. Paper presented at UNFPA-WHO/EURO-IPPF-Zhordania Institute From Abortion to Contraception, Tbilsi, 10–13 October: 1–7.

Bardon, Sylvie, Vignon, Françoise, Chalbos, Dany and Rochefort, Henri. (1985). RU 486, a progestin and glucocorticoid antagonist, inhibits the growth of breast cancer cells via the progesterone receptor. *Journal of Clinical Endocrinology and Metabolism 60*: 692–697.

Bart, Pauline. (1987). Seizing the Means of Reproduction: An Illegal Feminist Abortion Collective – How and Why it Worked. *Qualitative Sociology 10* (4): 339–357.

Baulieu, Etienne-Emile and Segal, Sheldon (Eds.). (1985). *The Antiprogestin Steroid RU 486 and Human Fertility Control.* Plenum Press: New York.

Baulieu, Etienne-Emile. (1985). RU 486: An Antiprogestin Steroid with Contragestive Activity in Women. In: Baulieu, Etienne-Emile and Segal, Sheldon (Eds.) *The Antiprogestin Steroid RU 486 and Human Fertility Control,* Plenum Press: New York: 1–27.

Baulieu, Etienne-Emile. (1988a). Contragestion with RU 486: A new approach to postovulatory fertility control. *Acta Obstetrica Gynecologica Scandinavica Supplement: 149:* 5–8.

Baulieu, Etienne-Emile. (1988b). A novel approach to human fertility control: contragestion by the anti-progesterone RU 486. *European Journal of Gynecology and Reproductive Biology 28:* 125–132.

Baulieu, Etienne-Emile. (1989a). RU-486 as an antiprogesterone steroid. The *Journal of the American Medical Association 262:* 1808–1814.

Baulieu, Etienne-Emile. (1989b). Contragestion and other clinical applications of RU 486, an antiprogesterone at the receptor. *Science 245:* 1351–1357.

Berer, Marge. (1988). RU 486 – News and Research. Women's Global Network for Reproductive Rights, *Newsletter* (Jan–Aug.): 21–22.

Berer, Marge. (1989). Report of a workshop on RU 486. Women's Global Network for Reproductive Rights, *Newsletter* (April–June): 2–3.

Bertagna, Xavier, Bertagna, Christine, Luton, Jean-Pierre, Husson, Marc and Girard, François. (1984). The new steroid analog RU 486 inhibits glucocorticoid action in man. *Journal of Clinical Endocrinology and Metabolism 59:* 25–28.

Bertagna, Xavier, Bertagna, Christine, Laudat, Marie-Helene, Husson, Jean-Marc, Girard, Francois and Luton, Jean-Pierre. (1986). Pituitary-adrenal response to the antiglucocorticoid action of RU 486 in Cushing's syndrome. *Journal of Clinical Endocrinology and Metabolism 63:* 639–643.

Bischof, P., Sizonenko, M.T. and Herrmann, W.L. (1986). Trophoblastic and decidual response to RU 486: effects on human chorionic gonadotrophin, human placental lactogen, prolactin and pregnancy-associated plasma protein-A production *in vitro*. *Human Reproduction 1*: 3–6.

Blankenstein, M.A., Van't Verlaat, J.W. and Croughs, R.J.M. (1989). Hormone dependency of meningiomas. *The Lancet i*: 1381–1382.

Bygdeman, Marc and Swahn, Marja-Liisa. (1985). Progesterone receptor blockage: Effect on uterine contractility and early pregnancy. *Contraception 32*: 45–51.

Bygdeman, Marc and Swahn, Marja-Liisa. (1989). Prostaglandins and antiprogestins. *Acta Obstetrica et Gynecologica Scandinavica Supplement 149*: 13–18.

Bygdeman, Marc, Christensen, Niels and Green, Krister. (1983). Clinical experience with selected prostaglandin analogues in obstetrics and gynaecology. In: *Cervagem. A new prostaglandin in obstetrics and gynaecology*. Sultan M.M. Karim (Ed.), MTP Press: Lancaster, Boston, The Hague: 63–76.

Cafarella, Jane (1991, 20 February). Should we swallow this pill? *The Age*, Melbourne: 16.

Cameron, I.T. and Baird, David, T. (1984). The use of 16,16 dimethyl-trans-δ^2-prostaglandin E_1 methyl ester (gemeprost) vaginal pessaries for the termination of pregnancy in the early second trimester. A comparison with extra-amniotic prostaglandin E_2. *British Journal of Obstetrics and Gynaecology 91*: 1136–1140.

Cameron, I.T., Michie, A.F. and Baird, David T. (1986). Therapeutic abortion in early pregnancy with antiprogestogen RU 486 alone or in combination with prostaglandin analogue (Gemeprost). *Contraception 34*: 459–469.

Cameron, I.T. and Baird, David T. (1988). Early pregnancy termination: a comparison between vacuum aspiration and medical abortion using prostaglandin (16,16 dimethyl-trans-δ^2-PGE$_1$ methyl ester) or the antiprogestogen RU 486. *British*

Journal of Obstetrics and Gynaecology 95: 271–276.

Caro, Denise. (1990, 23 May). Des médecins des centres d'IVG prennent la défense du RU 486. *Le Quotidien du Médecin* No. 4533: 10.

Cates, Willard and Jordaan, Harold V.F. (1979). Sudden collapse and death of women obtaining abortions induced with prostaglandin $F_{2\alpha}$. *American Journal of Obstetrics and Gynecology* 133: 398–400.

Cates, Willard, Grimes, David A., Haber. Richard J. and Tyler, Carl W. (1977). Abortion deaths associated with the use of prostaglandin $F_{2\alpha}$. *American Journal of Obstetrics and Gynecology* 127: 219–222.

Cekan, Sten, Aedo, Ana-Rosa, Segersteen, Eva, van Look, Paul, Messinis, Ioannis and Templeton, Allan. (1988). Levels of the antiprogestin RU 486 and its metabolites in human blood and follicular fluid following oral administration of a single dose. *Human Reproduction* 4: 131–135.

Chapman, Fern. (1989, 3 October). The Politics of the Abortion Pill. *Washington Post*: 11–13.

Chavkin, Wendy and Rosenfield, Allan. (1990). A chill wind blows: Webster, obstetrics, and the health of women. *American Journal of Obstetrics and Gynecology* 163: 450–452.

Clement, Connie. (1983). The Case for Lay Abortion. *Healthsharing*, Winter 1983, Toronto, Canada: 9–14.

Coles, Peter. (1989). RU 486 still troubled. *Nature 340*: 6.

Collins, Francis S. and Mahoney, Maurice J. (1983). Hydrocephalus and abnormal digits after failed first trimester abortion attempt. *Journal of Pediatrics 102*: 620–621.

Collins, R.L. and Hodgen, G.D. (1986). Blockade of the spontaneous midcycle gonadotropin surge in monkeys by RU 486: A progesterone antagonist or agonist? *Journal of Clinical Endocrinology and Metabolism 63*: 1270.

Connexions. (1989). RU 486: Revolutionary Discovery? Oakland, California: 15.

Coney, Sandra. (1990a, 26 November). RU 486 abortion drug. *The Dominion* (New Zealand): 11.

Coney, Sandra. (1990b, 27 November). A new age or a death drug? *The Herald* (New Zealand): 3.

Couzinet, Béatrice, Le Strat, Nelly, Ulmann, André, Baulieu, Etienne Emile and Schaison, Gilbert. (1986). Termination of early pregnancy by the progesterone antagonist RU 486 (Mifepristone). *The New England Journal of Medicine 315*: 1565–1570.

Couzinet, Béatrice, and Schaison, Gilbert (1988). Mifegyne (Mifepristone), a new antiprogestagen with potential therapeutic use in human fertility control. *Drugs* 35: 187–191.

Couzinet, Béatrice, Le Strat, Nelly, Silvestre, Louise and Schaison, Gilbert. (1990). Late luteal administration of the antiprogesterone RU 486* in normal women: effects on the menstrual cycle events and fertility control in a long-term study. *Fertility and Sterility 54* (6): 1039–1044.

Crooij, Marinus J., de Nooyer, Coenraad C.A., Rao, Ramanath, Berends, Gerrit T., Gooren, Louis J.G. and Janssens, Jannes. (1988). Termination of early pregnancy by the 3ß-hydroxysteroid dehydrogenase inhibitor epostane. *The New England Journal of Medicine 319*: 813–817.

Crowley, William. (1986). Progesterone antagonism. *The New England Journal of Medicine 315* (25): 1607–1608.

Csapo, Arpad I., Pulkkinen, Martti O. and Weist, W.G. (1973). Effects of lutectomy and progesterone replacement therapy in early pregnant patients. *American Journal of Obstetrics and Gynecology 115*: 759–765.

Csapo, Arpad I., Pulkkinen, Martti O., Ruttner, B., Sauvage, J.P. and Weist, W.G. (1972). The significance of the human corpus luteum in pregnancy maintenance. *American Journal of Obstetrics and Gynecology 112*: 1061–1067.

Csapo. Arpad I., Sauvage, J.P. and Weist, W.G. (1971). The efficacy and acceptability of intravenously administered prostaglandin $F_{2\alpha}$ as an abortifacient. *American Journal of*

Obstetrics and Gynecology 111: 1059–1063.

Das, Chandra and Catt, Kevin J. (1987). Antifertility actions of the progesterone antagonist RU 486 include direct inhibition of placental hormone secretion. *The Lancet ii* (12 September): 599–661.

de la Fuente, Martha. (1989). Letter to the Editor. Women's Global Network for Reproductive Rights, *Newsletter* (Oct/Dec) *31*: 3–4.

Delaney, Anne. (1990, 19 November). The Health Report. Radio National, Australia.

Delaney, Anne. (1991, 22 April). The Health Report. Radio National, Australia.

Department of Health, Education and Welfare. Public Health Service. National Institute of Health, USA. (1969). Request for proposals REP, Council for Population Control–69–1.

Deraedt, Roger, Bonnat, Claude, Busigny, Monique, Chatelet, Pierre, Cousty, Cristian, Mouren, Michel, Philibert, Daniel, Pottier, Jacques and Salmon, Jean. (1985). Pharmacokinetics of RU 486. In: *The Antiprogestin Steroid RU 486 and Human Fertility Control* edited by E.-E. Baulieu and S. Segal. Plenum Press: New York: 103–122.

Dietl, J. and Lippert, T.H. (1990). Critical comments on the treatment of tubal pregnancy with prostaglandins. *American Journal of Obstetrics and Gynecology 163*: 707.

Di Francesco, P., Pica, Francesca, Tubaro, E., Favalli, C. and Goraci, E. (1990). Inhibitory effects of cocaine on the cellular immune response in normal mice. *Abstract Book, 7th International Conference on Prostaglandins and Related Compounds*, May 28–June 1: 336.

Di Mattina M., Loriaux, D.L., Albertson, B.D., Falk, R.J. and Tyson, V. (1987). Effect of the antiprogestagen mifepristone on human ovarian steroidogenesis. *Fertility and Sterility 48*: 229–233.

Dorozynski, Alexander. (1988). Tempest in a pill box. *British Journal of Medicine 297*: 1291–1292.

Dumble, Lynette J. (1991). Current concerns for chemical abortion. *Proceedings* . Healthsharing Women Conference, Women and Surgery, September 1990, Melbourne (in press).

Elger, Walter, Qing, Shi Shao, Fahnrich, M., Beier, S., Chwalisz, Krzysztof, Henderson, D., Neef, G. and Rohde, R. (1987). The mechanism of action of new antiprogestins. In: *Fertility Regulation Today and Tomorrow*, edited by E. Diczfalusy and Marc Bygdeman, Raven Press: New York: 75–94.

Elze, Diane. (1988). Underground Abortion Remembered: Part II. *Soujorner: The Women's Forum*, May: 12–13.

Emanzipation. RU 486 – eine Wahl, die keine ist. (Jan/Feb) Basle, Switzerland: 12.

Euler, A.R., Leodolter, S., Huber, J., Lookabaugh, J., Burns, M.D., Phan, T.D., Wood, D.R., Bogaerts, H. and Kitt, M., (1989). Arbaprostil's [15 (R)-15-methyl PGE_2] Effects on Intrauterine Pressure in the Nonpregnant and Pregnant Human Female – A Report of Four Clinical Trials. *Prostaglandins Leukotrienes and Essential Fatty Acids, 38*: 91–98.

Ewing, Tania. (1990). Doubts over Abortion Pill. *Medical Observer* (Australia). 20 July–2 August: 1.

Fidler, Megan. (1991). RU 486 the new French Letter. *Broadsheet* Jan/Feb 1991: 27–29.

Frydman, René, Taylor, Sabine and Ulmann, André. (1985). Transplacental passage of Mifepristone. *The Lancet ii*: 1252.

Gaillard, R.D., Riondel, A., Muller, A.F., Herrmann, W. and Baulieu, E.E. (1984). RU 486: A steroid with anti-glucocortisteroid activity that only disinhibits the human pituitary-adrenal system at a specific time of day. *Proc. Natl. Acad. Sci 81*, 3879–3882.

Gao Ji, Qiao Gen-Mei, Wu Yu-Ming, Wu Muzh-En, Zheng Shu-Rong, Han Zhi-Bai, Fan Huimin, Yao Guang-Zhen, Meng Ung, Dubois, Catherine, Ulmann, André and Baulieu, Etienne-Emile. (1988). Pregnancy interruption with RU 486 in combination with dl-15-methyl-prostaglandin-$F_{2\alpha}$-methyl ester: the Chinese experience. *Contraception 38*: 675–683.

Gardner, Marilyn. (1989, 5 December). RU 486 – New technology, old choices. *The Christian Science Monitor*: 6.

Gillies, Fiona. (1990, 5 August). Reynolds appeals for new abortion pill tets. *The Sunday Herald,* Melbourne: 7.

Goodman, Ellen. (1989, 17 July). Moral Property. *The Boston Globe*: 11.

Goodman, Ellen. (1990, 1 July). Year after Webster. *The Boston Globe*: 1.

Gordon, Linda. (1976). *Woman's Body, Woman's Right.* Grossman Publishers: New York.

Gravanis, A., Schaison, G., George, M., de Brux, J., Satyaswaroop, P.G., Baulieu, E.E. and Robel, P. (1985). Endometrial and pituitary responses to the steroidal antiprogestin RU 486 in postmenopausal women. *Journal of Clinical Endocrinology and Metabolism 60*: 156–163.

Grimes, David A., Mishell, Daniel R., Shoupe, Donna and Lacarra, Maria. (1988). Early abortion with a single dose of the antiprogestin RU-486. *American Journal of Obstetrics and Gynecology 158*: 1307–1312.

Grimes, David A., Berstein, Leslie, Lacarra, Maria, Shoupe, Donna and Mishell, Daniel R. (1990). Predictors of failed attempted abortion with the antiprogestin mifepristone (RU 486). *American Journal of Obstetrics and Gynecology 162*: 910–917.

Gruppe Prostaglandine. (1981). *Prostaglandine beim Schwangerschaftsabbruch. Wem nützen sie?* Hamburg Selbstverlag.

Healy, David L. and Hodgen, Gary D. (1985). Non-human primate studies with RU 486. In: *The Antiprogestin Steroid RU 486 and Human Fertility Control,* edited by E.-E. Baulieu and S. Segal. Plenum Press: New York: 127–140.

Heikinheimo, Oskari, Teveilin, Marjatta, Shoupe, Donna, Croxatto, Horacio and Lahteenmaki, Pekka. (1986). Quantitation of RU 486 in human plasma by HPLC and RIA after column chromatography. *Contraception 34*: 613–624.

Henrion, R. (1989). RU 486 abortions. *Nature 338*: 110.

Herman, Robin. (1989, 3 October). The politics of the abortion pill. *Washington Post*: 12.

Herrmann, W.L., Wyss, Rolf, Riondel, A., Philibert, Daniel, Teutsch, Georges, Sakiz, Eduord and Baulieu, Etienne-Emile. (1982). Effet d'un stéroide antiprogesterone chez la femme: interruption du cycle menstruel et de la grossesse au début. *C R Acad Sci Paris 294*: 933–938.

Hill, Nicholas, Ferguson, Jane, and MacKenzie I.Z. (1990a). The efficacy of oral Mifepristone (RU 38,486) with a prostaglandin E_1 analog vaginal pessary for the termination of early pregnancy: Complications and patient acceptability. *American Journal of Obstetrics and Gynecology 162*: 414–417.

Hill, Nicholas C.W. and MacKenzie, Ian Z. (1990b). Early termination of pregnancy: Medical induction with prostaglandins versus surgical abortion under local anaesthetic. *International Journal of Gynecology and Obstetrics 32*: 269–274.

Hills, Ben. (1988, 21 June). Abortion pill trials called off. *The Herald*, Melbourne: 3.

Hodgen, Gary D. (1985). Pregnancy prevention by intravaginal delivery of progesterone antagonist: RU486 tampon for menstrual induction and absorption. *Fertility and Sterility 44*: 263–267.

Hughes, Sylvia. (1990, 5 May). Anti-abortionists renew attack on French pill. *New Scientist*: 3.

Husslein, P., Fitz, R., Pateisky, N. and Egarter, C. (1989). Prostaglandin injection for termination of tubal pregnancy: preliminary results. *American Journal of Perinatology 6*: 117–120.

Hynes, H. Patricia. (1990). Reconstructing Babylon: Women and Appropriate Technology. Keynote Address given at Nordic Conference on Women, Environment, and Development. Norwegian Research Council for Science and the Humanities, the Secretariat for Women and Research. Oslo, 13–15 November: 1–38.

Ince, Susan. (1991). The Trouble with RU 486. *Vogue* (July): 88–90.

Ingvardsen, A. and Eriksen, T. (1979). Cervical rupture following prostaglandin-induced mid-trimester abortion. *Ugeskr Laeger 141*: 3531.

ISIS Women's Health Journal. (1989). RU 486 – Another Fake Miracle? No. 11–12: 32

ISIS Women's Health Journal. (1990). France to Subsidize Abortion Pill Use. No.18: 8.

Jerve, Fridtjof, Fylling, Petter and Stenby, Steinar. (1979). Rupture of the uterus following treatment with 16-16-dimethyl E_2 prostaglandin vagitories. *Prostaglandins, 17*: 121–123.

Jost, A. (1986). Animal reproduction–new data on the hormonal requirement of the pregnant rabbit; partial pregnancies and fetal abnormalities resulting from a treatment with a hormonal antagonist given at sub-abortive dosage. *CR Acad. Sci. III 7*: 281–84.

Juneja, Subhash C. and Dodson, Melvin G. (1990). *In vitro* effect of RU 486 on sperm-egg interaction in mice. *American Journal of Obstetrics and Gynecology 163*: 216–221.

Kafrissen, Michael E. (1990). Prevention of cardiovascular risk in women. *Acta Obstetrica Gynecologica Scandinavica Supplement 152*: 13–20.

Kajanoja, Pauli (1983). Induction of Abortion by Prostaglandins in the Second Trimester of Pregnancy. *Acta Obstetrica et Gynecologica Scandinavica Supplement 113*: 145–151.

Kami, Myriam. (1990, 20 April). RU 486: la tolérance, nouveau sujet de controverse. *Le Quotidien du Médecin* No. 4512: 9.

Karim, Sultan M.M. (Ed.). (1983). *Cervagem: A New Prostaglandin in Obstetrics and Gynaecology.* MTP Press: Lancaster, Boston, The Hague.

Karim, Sultan M.M. (1983). Clinical applications of prostaglandins in obstetrics and gynaecology. In: *Cervagem: A New Prostaglandin in Obstetrics and Gynaecology,* edited by Sultan M.M. Karim. MTP Press: Lancaster: 15–34.

Karim, Sultan M.M. and Filshie, G.M. (1970). Therapeutic

abortion using prostaglandin $F_{2\alpha}$. *The Lancet, i*: 157–159.

Kekkonen, Raimo, Alfthan, Henrik, Haukkamaa, Maija, Heikinheimo, Oskari, Luukkainen, Tapani, and Lahteenmaki, Pekka. (1990). Interference with ovulation by sequential treatment with the antiprogesterone RU 486 and synthetic progestin. *Fertility and Sterility 53*: 747–750.

Kingman, Sharon. (1989, 4 November). Drug company holds back abortion pill. *New Scientist*: 4.

Klein, Renate/Rowland Robyn. (1988). Women as test-sites for fertility drugs: Clomiphene citrate and hormonal cocktails. *Reproductive and Genetic Engineering: Journal of International Feminist Analysis 1*(3): 251–274.

Klein, Renate. (1991). RU 486 A New Miracle Drug! Or is it? *Inkwell* No. 1 (Jan/Feb) Canberra: 17–19.

Kleinman, Ronald L. (Ed.) (1990). *Hormonal Contraception.* International Planned Parenthood Federation: London.

Kovacs, L., Sas, M., Resch, B.A., Ugocsai, G., Swahn, Marja-Liisa, Bygdeman, Marc and Rowe, P.J. (1984). Termination of early pregnancy by RU 486 – an antiprogestational compound. *Contraception 29: 399–410.*

Krier, Ann Beth. (1990, 22 April). Dr. Grimes' bitter pill. *Los Angeles Times*: E1, E12, E13 and E14.

Lange, Aksel P. (1983). Prostaglandins as abortifacients in Denmark. *Acta Obstetrica et Gynecologica Scandinavica Supplement 113*: 117–124.

La Révue Prescrire. (1990). Médicament à délivrance particulière: Myfégyne. (July/August) *10* (98): 286–288.

Laue, Luisa, Lotze, Michael T., Chrousos, George P., Barnes, Kevin, Loriaux, Lynn and Fleisher, Thomas A. (1990). Effect of Chronic Treatment with the Glucocorticoid Antagonist RU 486 in Man: Toxicity, Immunological, and Hormonal Aspects. *Journal of Clinical Endocrinology and Metabolism 71* (6): 1474–1480.

Le Grand, Amanda. (1990). Medical and users' aspects of RU 486 with particular emphasis on its use in Third World countries. In: *WEMOS Proceedings*: 19–28.

Lee, Min-Wei. (1990, 28 June). AMA urges U.S. test of 'abortion pill'. *Chicago Tribune:* 1–2.

Lépinay, Michel. (1982, 22 April). Seconde révolution contraceptive: La pilule de fin de cycle. *Libération:* 2.

Levin, Jay H., Lacarra, Maria, d'Ablaing, Gerrit, Grimes, David A. and Vermesh, Michael. (1990). Mifepristone (RU 486) failure in an ovarian heterotopic pregnancy. *American Journal of Obstetrics and Gynecology 163*: 543–544.

Li, Tin-Chiu, Dockery, Peter, Thomas, Peter, Rogers, Andrew W., Lenton, Elizabeth A. and Cooke, Ian D. (1988). The effects of progesterone receptor blockade in the luteal phase of normal fertile women. *Fertility and Sterility 50*: 732–742.

Lim, B.H., Lees, D.A.R., Bjornsson, S., Lunan, C.B., Cohn, M.R., Stewart, P. and Davey, A.(1990). Normal development after exposure to mifepristone in early pregnancy. *The Lancet* (28 July) *336*: 257–258.

Los Angeles Times. (1990, 6 May). Letters in View. Pros and Cons of Dr. Grimes' 'bitter pill': E 14 and 20.

Luukkainen, Tapani, Heikinheimo, Oskari, Haukkamaa, Maija and Lahteenmaki, Pekka. (1988). Inhibition of folliculogenesis and ovulation by the antiprogesterone RU 486. *Fertility and Sterility 49*: 961–963.

MacKinnon, Catharine. (1987). Privacy v. Equality: Beyond Roe v. Wade. In: *Feminism Unmodified. Discourses on Life and Law.* Harvard University Press: Cambridge, USA: 93–102.

Maria, Bernard, Stampf, Françoise, Goepp, Anne and Ulmann, André. (1988). Termination of early pregnancy by a single dose of mifepristone (RU 486), a progesterone antagonist. *European Journal of Obstetrics and Gynecology and Reproductive Biology 28*: 249–255.

McIntosh, Philip. (1990, 24 July). Professor urges introduction of abortion pill. *The Age*: 5.

Messinis, Ioannis E. and Templeton, Allan. (1988). The effect of the antiprogestin mifepristone (RU 486) on maturation and *in-vitro* fertilization of human oocytes. *British Journal of Obstetrics and Gynaecology 95*: 592–595.

Meyer, Elsbeth, von Paczensky, Susanne and Sadrozinski, Renate. (1990). *'Das hätte nicht noch mal passieren dürfen!' Wiederholte Schwangerschaftsabbrüche und was dahintersteckt.* Fischer Verlag: Frankfurt.

Moore, Rosemary. (1990). RU 486 – A boon drug? *Healthsharing Women*, Melbourne (September/October): 5–8.

Moran, Mark, Mozes, Martin F., Maddux, Michael S., Veremis, Susan., Bartkus, Cynthia, Ketal, Beverly, Pollak, Raymond, Wallemark, Carl and Jonasson, Olga. (1990). Prevention of acute graft rejection by the prostaglandin E1 analogue Misoprostol in renal-transplant recipients treated with cyclosporine and prednisone. *The New England Journal of Medicine 322*: 1183–1188.

National Women's Health Network. (1989). *Abortion Then and Now: Creative Responses to Restricted Access.* 1352 G Street, N.W. Washington DC 20005, USA.

Nau, Jean-Yves. (1990, 19 August). Drug firm defends marketing strategy on abortion pill. *Guardian Weekly*: 16.

Nau, Jean-Ives and Franck Nouchi. (1988, 30–31 October). La pilule abortive au nom de la loi. *Le Monde*: 9.

Newsletter. (1990). Human embryology and fertilisation bill. Women's Health and Reproductive Rights Centre, London, UK: 15–16.

Newztel Log. (1990, 20 November). Good Morning NZ. Radio New Zealand (Transcript).

Nieman, Lynnette K., Chrousos, George P., Kellner, Charles, Spitz, Irving M., Nisula, Bruce C., Cutler, Gordon B., Merriam, George R., Bardin, C. Wayne and Loriaux, D. Lynn. (1985). Successful treatment of Cushing's syndrome with the glucocorticoid antagonist RU 486. *Journal of Clinical Endocrinology and Metabolism 61*: 536–540.

Nieman, Lynnette K. and Loriaux, D. Lynn. (1988). The use of anti-progesterones as a medical IUD. *Bailliere's Clinical Obstetrics and Gynaecology 2*: 609–615.

Nissim, Rina. (1989). Letter to the Editor. Women's Global Network for Reproductive Rights *Newsletter 31* (Oct–Dec): 5.

Nouchi, Franck. (1988, 28 October). Mgr Lustinger estime que le retrait du RU 486 est dû à des problèmes de 'pharma-covigilance'. *Le Monde*: 12.

Ob. Gyn. News. (1989). RU 486 and progestin combination could yield estrogen-free OC. *24* (8): 15, 38.

Ob. Gyn. News. (1989). RU 486 may have many uses if it can survive the abortion war. *24* (14): 1

Odlind, Viveca and Birgerson, Lars. (1987). Interruption of early gestation with Antiprogestins. In: *Fertility Regulation Today and Tomorrow*, edited by E. Diczfalusy and M. Bygdeman, Raven Press, New York: 95–104.

Ortmann, Olaf, Emons, Gunter, Knuppen, Rudolf and Catt, Kevin J. (1989). Inhibitory effects of the antiprogestin, RU 486, on progesterone actions and luteinizing hormone secretion in pituitary gonadotrophs. *Journal of Steroid Biochemistry 32*: 291–297.

Parinaud, Jean, Perret Bertrand, Ribbes, Huguette, Vieitez, Gerard and Baulieu, Etienne-Emile. (1990). Effects of RU 486 on Progesterone Secretion by Human Preovulatory Granulosa Cells in Culture. *Journal of Clinical Endocrinology and Metabolism 70* (6): 1534–1537

Permezel, M. (1990). The antiprogesterone steroid, RU 486 (Mifepristone). *Australian and New Zealand Journal of Obstetrics and Gynaecology 30*: 77–80.

Perspectives in Family Planning. (1988). New treatment to end early pregnancy found to be safe and effective. Digest Section (Sept/Oct): 241.

Phillips, Calbert I., Gore, Sheila M., Green, Keith, Cullen, Patricia M. and Campbell, Marion. (1984). Eye drops of RU 486-6, a periphereal steroid blocker, lower intra-ocular pressure in rabbits. *The Lancet i:* 767–768.

Quinn, M.A. and Murphy, A.J. (1981). Fetal death following extra-amniotic prostaglandin gel: Report of two cases. *British Journal of Obstetrics and Gynaecology 88*: 650–651.

Rauch, Judith. (1990). Abtreibungspille. *Emma* (March): 6.

Raymond, Janice G. (1991). RU 486 A Medical Miracle? *Spare Rib* (UK) February: 34–37.

Redgrave, Nicholas G., Dumble, Lynette J., Pollak, Raymond, Ruwart, Mary J. and Clunie, Gordon J.A. (1991a). An *in vitro* comparison of the immunosuppressive potential of synthetic prostaglandin analogues. *Transplantation Proceedings 23*: 346–347.

Redgrave, Nicholas G., Dumble, Lynette J., Francis, David M.A., Plenter, Robert, Ruwart, Mary J., Birchall, Ian and Clunie, Gordon J.A. (1991b). Synergistic prolongation of rabbit renal allograft survival by cyclosporine and a prostacyclin analogue, U-62840. *Transplantation Proceedings* (in press).

Riding, Alan. (1990, 29 July). Abortion politics are said to hinder use of French pill. *New York Times*: A1 and A15.

Riding, Alan. (1991, 10 April). Frenchwoman's death tied to the use of abortion pill. *New York Times*: A10.

Rodger, Mary W. and Baird, David T. (1987). Induction of therapeutic abortion in early pregnancy with mifepristone in combination with prostaglandin pessary. *The Lancet* (December 19): 1415–1418.

Rodger, Mary W. and Baird, David T. (1989). Blood loss following a prostaglandin analogue (Gemeprost). *Contraception 40*: 439–447.

Rosén, Anne-Sofie, Nystedt, Lars, Bygdeman, Marc and Lundstrom, Viveca. (1979). Acceptability of a nonsurgical method to terminate very early pregnancy in comparison to vacuum aspiration. *Contraception 19*: 107–117.

Rothman, Lorraine. (1978). Menstrual Extraction Procedures. *Quest* 4(3): 44–48.

Sadrozinski, Renate. (1990). *Ambulanter Schwangerschaftsabbruch*

– *Eine Studie der Familienplanungszentren.* Unpublished study.

Sapsted, Anne-Marie. (1991, 6 January). Abortion: The new pill. *Sunday Times Magazine* (UK): 40–42.

Schneider, Martin, R., Michna, Horst, Nishino Yukishige, Neef, Günter and El Etreby, Fathy M. (1990). Tumor-Inhibiting Potential of ZK 112.993, a New Progesterone Antagonist, in Hormone-Sensitive, Experimental Rodent and Human Mammary Tumors. *Anticancer Research 10*: 683–688.

Schönhöfer, Peter S. (1991). Brazil: Misuse of misoprostol as an abortifacient may induce malformations. *The Lancet 337*: 1534–1535.

Schreiber, James R., Hsueh, Aaron J.W. and Baulieu, E.E. (1983). Binding of the anti-progestin RU-486 to rat ovary steroid receptors. *Contraception 28*: 77–81.

Secher, N.J., Thayssen, P, Arnsbo, P. and Olsen, J. (1982). Effect of prostaglandin E2 and F2 on the systemic and pulmonary circulation in pregnant anaesthetized women. *Acta Obstetrica et Gynecologica Scandinavica 63*: 213–218.

Segal, Sheldon J. (1990). Mifepristone (RU 486). *The New England Journal of Medicine 322*: 691–693.

Shi Wenliang and Zhu Pengdi. (1990). Autoradiographic localization of [3H]RU 486 and [3H] progesterone in the uterus, pituitary and hypothalamus of the rat. *Human Reproduction 5* (2): 123–127.

Shoupe, Donna, Mishell, Daniel R., Page, Mary Alice, Madkour, Hosam, Spitz, Irving M. and Lobo, Rogerio A. (1987). Effects of the antiprogesterone RU 486 in normal women. II. Administration in the late follicular phase. *American Journal of Obstetrics and Gynecology 157*: 1421–1426.

Silvestre, Louise, Dubois, Catherine, Renault, Maguy, Rezvani, Yvonne, Baulieu, Etienne-Emile and Ulmann, André. (1990). Voluntary interruption of pregnancy with Mifepristone (RU 486) and a prostaglandin analogue. *The New England Journal of Medicine 322*: 645–648.

Simmons, Katie and Savage, Wendy. (1984). Neonatal death

associated with induction of labour with intravaginal prostaglandin E2. *British Journal of Obstetrics and Gynaecology 91*: 598–599.

Simons, Marlise. (1988, 28 October). A medical outcry greets suspension of abortion pill. *The New York Times*: A1 and A8.

Sitruk-Ware, R., Bilaud, L., Mowszowicz, I., Yaneva, H., Mauvais-Jarvis, P., Bardin, C.W. and Spitz, I.M. (1985). The use of RU 486 as an abortifacient in early pregnancy. In: *The Antiprogestin Steroid RU 486 and Human Fertility Control*, edited by E.-E. Baulieu and S. Segal. Plenum Press: New York: 243–247.

Sitruk-Ware, Regine, Thalabard, Jean-Christophe, De Plunkett, Tu Lan, Lewin, Fanny, Epelboin, Sylvie, Mowszowicz, Irene, Yaneva, Halina, Tournaire, Michel, Chavinie, Jacques, Mauvais-Jarvis, Pierre and Spitz, Irving. (1990). The use of the antiprogestin RU486 (mifepristone) as an abortifacient in early pregnancy – clinical and pathological findings; predictive factors for efficacy. *Contraception 41*: 221–243.

Somell, Christina and Ölund, Anders. (1990). Induction of abortion in early pregnancy with mifepristone. *Gynecologic and Obstetric Investigations 29*: 13–15.

Sontag, S.J., Mazure, P. A., Pontes, J.F., Beker, S.G. and Dajani, E.Z. (1985). Misoprostol in the treatment of duodenal ulcer. A multicenter double-blind placebo-controlled study. *Digestive Diseases and Sciences 30*: 159S–163S.

Stuenkel, Cynthia A., Garzo, V. Gabriel, Morris, Stephen, Liu, James H. and Yen, Samuel S.C. (1990). Effects of the antiprogesterone RU 486 in the early follicular phase of the menstrual cycle. *Fertility and Sterility 53*: 642–646.

Sunday Times Magazine (UK). (1988, 30 October). French Abortion Pill on Sale Here in 1990.

Swahn, Marja-Liisa and Bygdeman, Marc. (1987). Interruption of early gestation with prostaglandins and antiprogestin. In: *Fertility Regulation Today and Tomorrow*, edited by E. Diczfalusy and M. Bygdeman, Raven Press: New York: 109–118.

Swahn, Marja-Liisa and Bydgeman, Marc. (1989). Termination

of early pregnancy with RU 486 (Mifepristone) in combination with a prostaglandin analogue (Sulprostone). *Acta Obstetrica Gynecologica Scandinavica 68*: 293–300.

Swahn, Marja-Liisa, Gottlieb, C., Green, Krister and Bygdeman, Marc. (1990). Oral administration of RU 486 and 9-methylene PGE$_2$ for termination of early pregnancy. *Contraception 41*: 461–473.

The Feminist Majority Foundation (1990). RU 486 *Communiqué* (n.d; n.pp).

Tonti-Filippini, Nicholas. (1990). RU 486: Dispelling Some Myths. St. Vincent's Bioethics Centre, *Newsletter* (June) *8* (2): 11–14.

Ulmann, André, Dubois, Catherine and Philibert, Daniel. (1987). Fertility control with RU 486. *Hormone Research 28*: 274–278.

Ulmann, André, Teutsch, Georges and Philibert, Daniel. (1990). RU 486. *Scientific American 262*: 42–48.

UK Multicentre Trial. (1990). The efficacy and tolerance of mifepristone and prostaglandin in first trimester termination of pregnancy. *British Journal of Obstetrics and Gynaecology 97*: 480–486.

Urquhart, D. R., and Templeton, A. A. (1988). Acceptability of medical pregnancy termination. *The Lancet* (July 9): 106–107.

van Look, Paul, F.A. (1990). The use of RU 486 (mifepristone) as a medical abortifacient; current and future research needs. In: *WEMOS Proceedings*: 1–4

Van Santen, M.R. and Haspels, A.A. (1987). Interception IV: Failure of Mifepristone (RU 486) as a monthly contragestive, 'Lunarette'. *Contraception 35*: 433–439.

Vervest, Harry A.M. and Haspels, Ary A. (1985). Preliminary results with the antiprogestational compound RU-486 (mifepristone) for interruption of early pregnancy. *Fertility and Sterility 44*: 627–632.

Vigy, Monique. (1991, 29 January). RU 486: l' 'excès du pouvoir' du ministre. *Le Figaro*: 18.

Vincent, R. Judith. (1990). RU 486: The miracle abortion?

Sojourner: The Women's Forum (March): 11H.

Wainer, Jo (1991). RU486: Another View. *Inkwell* No 1 (Jan/Feb) Canberra: 19–20.

Waltman, Richard, Tricorni, Vincent and Palay, Aravind. (1973). Aspirin and indomethacin: Effect on installation/abortion time of mid-trimester hypertonic saline induced abortions. *Prostaglandins 3*: 47–58.

WEMOS, Women and Pharmaceuticals. (1990). *Proceedings, Seminar on RU 486: The Abortion Pill.* Amsterdam, The Netherlands.

Wiederkehr, Julio C., Dumble, Lynette J., Pollak, Raymond and Moran, Mark. (1990). Immunosuppressive effect of Misoprostol: a new synthetic prostaglandin E1 analogue. *Australia and New Zealand Journal of Surgery 60*: 121–124.

Wolf, Jean Philippe, Hsiu, JG, Ulman André, Baulieu Etienne-Emile and Hodgen, Gary D. (1987). RU 486 blocks the mitogenic action of estrogen on the endometrium by a potent progesterone agonist effect. *Biology of Reproduction 36* (Suppl 1): 109.

Wolf, Jean Phillipe, Danforth, Douglas R., Ulmann, André, Baulieu, Etienne-Emile and Hodgen, Gary D. (1989). Contraceptive potential of RU 486 by ovulation inhibition: II. suppression of pituitary gonadotropin secretion *in vitro. Contraception 40*: 185–193.

Wolf, Jean Phillipe, Chillik, Claudio F., Dubois, Catherine, Ulmann, André, Baulieu, Etienne-Emile and Hodgen, Gary D. (1990). Tolerance of perinidatory primate embryos to RU 486 exposure *in vitro* and *in vivo. Contraception 41*: 85–92.

Wood, P.L., Burgess, S.P. and Dison, P. (1987). Growth retardation and fetal hydrocephalus developing after discontinuation of a mid-trimester termination procedure. Case report. *British Journal of Obstetrics and Gynaecology 94*: 372–374.

World Health Organization. (1972). *Report from Meetings of the Prostaglandin Steering Committee,* edited by Sune Bergström. Research and Training Centre on Human Reproduction,

Karolinska Institutet: Stockholm, Sweden.

World Health Organization. (1987). Menstrual regulation by intramuscular injections of 16-phenoxy-tetranor PGE₂ methyl sulfonylamide or vacuum aspiration. A randomized multicentre study. *British Journal of Obstetrics and Gynaecology, 94*: 949–956.

World Health Organization. (1989a). Termination of early human pregnancy with RU 486 (mifepristone) and the prostaglandin analogue sulprostone: a multi-centre, randomized comparison between two treatment regimens. *Human Reproduction 4* (6): 718–725.

World Health Organization. (1989b). Menstrual regulation by intramuscular injections of 16-phenoxy-tetranor PGE₂ methyl sulphonylamide (sulprostone). A multicentre study. *British Journal of Obstetrics and Gynaecology 96*: 207–212.

World Health Organization. (1990). The use of mifepristone (RU 486) for cervical preparation in first trimester pregnancy termination by vacuum aspiration. *British Journal of Obstetrics and Gynaecology 97*: 260–266.

Yang, Y.Q., and Wu, J.T. (1990). RU 486 interferes with egg transport and retards the *in vivo* and *in vitro* development of mouse embryos. *Contraception 41*: 551–556.

Zheng, Shu-rong. (1989). RU 486 (Mifepristone): Clinical trials in China. *Acta Obstetrica Gynecologica Scandinavica Supplement 149*: 19–23.

zur Nieden, Sabine. (1990). Diese Pille gibt Frauen Freiheit. *Emma* (June): 26–27.